KNACK
MAKE IT EASY

FIRST
AID

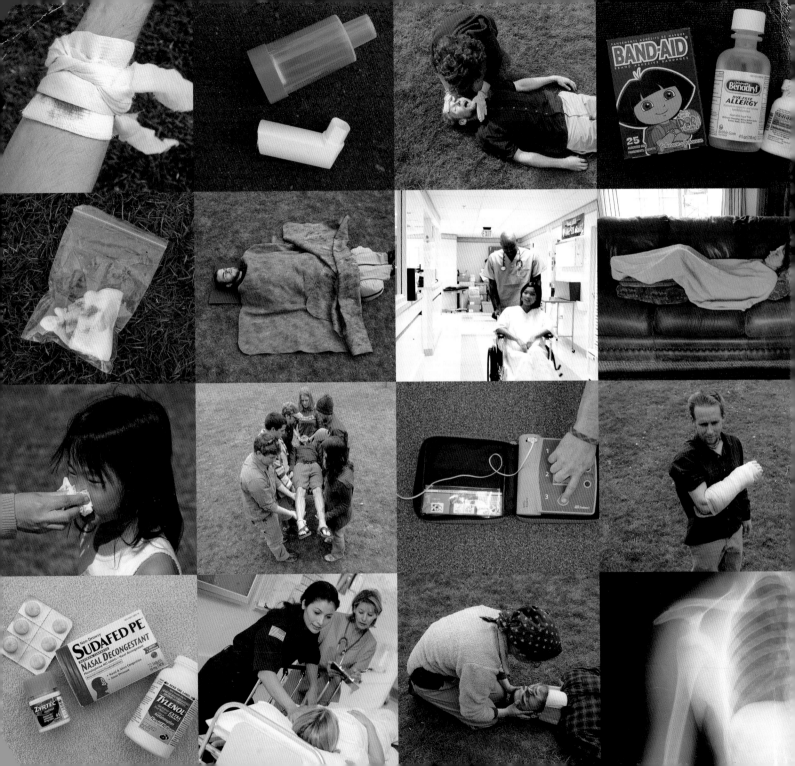

KNACK

FIRST AID

A Complete Illustrated Guide

BUCK TILTON

Photographs by Stephen Gorman and Eli Burakian

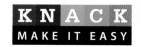

Guilford, Connecticut
An imprint of Globe Pequot Press

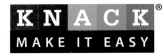

Editorial Director: Cynthia Hughes
Editor: Katie Benoit
Project Editor: Tracee Williams
Cover Design: Paul Beatrice, Bret Kerr
Interior Design: Paul Beatrice
Layout: Kevin Mak
Cover Photos by: Stephen Gorman and Eli Burakian
All interior photos by Stephen Gorman and Eli Burakian with the exception of p. 18 (right): © Axel Plessmann | Jupiter Images; p. 61 (left): © Distinctiveimages | Dreamstime.com; p. 116 (left): © ryasick | Shutterstock.com; p. 117 (left): © Jupiter Images; p. 133 (left): © Jupiter Images; p. 136 (left): © Paul-André Belle-Isle | Jupiter Images; p. 136 (right): © Jupiter Images; p. 139 (right): © Christine Kublanski | Jupiter Images; p. 142 (left): © Carmen Reed | Jupiter Images; p. 150 (right): © Christophe Testi | Jupiter Images; p. 158 (left): © Forest Woodward | Jupiter Images; p. 158 (right): © Elena Elisseeva | Jupiter Images; p. 162 (right): © Mads Frederiksen | Jupiter Images; p. 164 (right): © Andrew Hagen | Jupiter Images; p. 165 (left): © Christian Nasca | Jupiter Images; p. 166 (left): © Gene Lee | Jupiter Images; p. 168 (left): © Wojciech Wojcik | Dreamstime.com; p. 170 (right): © Lev Ezhov | Jupiter Images, p. 171 (left): © Sebastian Kaulitzki | Dreamstime.com; p. 172 (left): © Johnbell | Dreamstime.com; p. 172 (right): © Jake Holmes | istockphoto; p. 173 (left) © Darren Green | Dreamstime.com; p. 173 (right): © Dave Rodriguez | istockphoto; p. 174 (left): © Brian Chase | Shutterstock.com; p. 174 (right): © Clint Spencer | istockphoto; p. 175 (left): Courtesy of Joe Belnap, Big H Products, Inc.; p. 176 (right): © Nico Smit | Jupiter Images; p. 17 (left): © Dan Mccauley | Dreamstime.com; p. 178 (left): © Kobby Dagan | Dreamstime.com; p. 178 (right): © Gilles Decruyenaere | Dreamstime.com; p. 179 (left): © Kevin Herrin | istockphoto; p. 183 (left): © Aldo Murillo | Jupiter Images; p. 193 (right): © Monkey Business Images | Shutterstock.com; p. 194 (right): © Vlad Turchenko | Dreamstime.com; p. 195 (left): © 2009 Jupiterimages Corporation, a Getty Images company; p. 198 (right): © Vivid Pixels | Shutterstock.com; p. 197 (left): © richard churchill | Jupiter Images; p. 200 (left) Illustration by Robert L. Prince; p. 201 (right): Photographed by Carline Jean; p. 202 (left): © Marcin-linfernum | Shutterstock.com; p. 202 (right): © Jupiter Images; p. 203 (left): © Valentin Mosichev | Jupiter Images; p. 209 (right): Photographed by Sue Barr; p. 211 (Left): Photographed by Susana Bates; p. 212 (right): © Oleg Kozlov | Jupiter Images; p. 216 (left): © Lisa F. Young | Dreamstime.com; p. 217 (left): © Oscar Williams | Dreamstime.com; p. 218 (left): © Jose AS Reyes | Shutterstock.com; p. 219 (right): © Lisa F. Young | Shutterstock.com; p. 220 (left): © Zoom-zoom | Dreamstime.com; p. 221 (left): © delihayat | Shutterstock.com

Library of Congress Cataloging-in-Publication Data
Tilton, Buck.
  Knack first aid : a complete illustrated guide / Buck Tilton ; photographs by Stephen Gorman & Eli Burakian.
     p. cm.
  ISBN 978-1-59921-818-2
  1. First aid in illness and injury—Handbooks, manuals, etc. I. Gorman, Stephen, II. Burakian, Eli. III. Title. IV. Title: First aid.
  RC86.8.T554 2010
  616.02′52--dc22

                    2009043611

The following manufacturers/names appearing in *Knack First Aid* are trademarks:
BAND-AID®, Dramamine®, EpiPen®, Gamow®, SAM®, Twinject®

Printed in China
10 9 8 7 6 5 4 3 2 1

To my family—Kathleen, Amber, McKenzie, Zachary, and Bo Tilton—first, last, and all the in-between.

Acknowledgments

It is never, ever a one-person job. It isn't even a job that allows me to meet all the people who contribute time and talent. I know, and deeply appreciate, the people who were graciously bandaged, splinted, and made bloody as models for the photographs—Jess Crawford, Joe Denniston, Ben Doyle, Micah Loyd, Taylor Stilton, and Kathleen and Bo Tilton. I know some of the people at Adventure Medical Kits who generously donated first-aid supplies for the photographs. And I know some of the great folks at Globe Pequot Press, including the benevolent mastermind Maureen Graney, where all this originates and then finishes. "Thank you" to those known and unknown.

CONTENTS

INTRODUCTION

In case you start here—and some readers actually do start here, with the introduction—there are a few things you need to know. In case you come here later, I hope it's not too late.

First, first-aid books are not very much like cookbooks. If you want to make a fifteen-bean soup, pretty much everything you need to know about cooking fifteen-bean soup—the ingredients, the amounts of the ingredients, how and when to mix the ingredients, the temperature to cook at, how long to cook, and even the kind of pot to use—will be on one page. First-aid books do not work that way. If you are helping someone with a furiously bleeding laceration (Chapter 3), and that person also has a chest injury that is making it difficult to breathe (Chapter 5), you don't have time to flip back and forth between Chapters 3 and 5. If you want to be a good first-aid provider, you should sit down in a quiet spot, perhaps with a favored beverage, and read

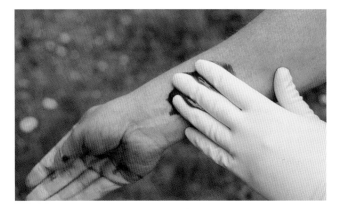

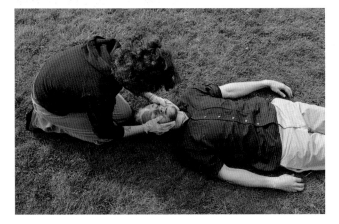

through this whole book, assimilating as much as possible before an emergency requiring your intervention arises.

Next, most books about first aid, and certainly this book about first aid, are progressive. What I mean by that is this: What you learn about in early chapters will help you understand, and, more importantly, understand what to do when you respond to emergencies covered in later chapters. For instance, if you have read the material in Chapter 1, you will probably be a better first-aid provider after you've read Chapters 5 and 8 than if you read Chapters 5 and 8 first. And even if that isn't true for you, you'll surely better understand Chapters 5 and 8 after you've read Chapter 1. That said, I have attempted to incorporate nuggets of information into many chapters that hopefully will remind you of information in previous chapters. My ultimate goal has been twofold: to help you be the best first-aid provider possible, and to help you remember that a person who needs first aid is a whole person and not just a broken arm or a mosquito bite.

Speaking of a "person," I have used the term "patient" hundreds of times in this book. I have been trained to refer to people requiring first aid as "patients," and I have come to appreciate the term. When I think of someone as my patient, even if I'm scrubbing an abrasion on the knee of one of my kids, it reminds me, as I think it reminds physicians, that this person deserves my best. It also reminds me that I need to be patient. And anyway "patient" is a respectful term.

You have some interest, or else you would not have continued to read to this point. So, allow me to ask you, "What is first aid?" Your answers might range from finding the box of Band-Aids to dropping to your knees to perform CPR to whipping out your cell phone to dial 911—and all those answers are correct. There is, in other words, no simple response to the question.

Someone might be injured, or someone might be sick, and you might be the first person there who can help. The

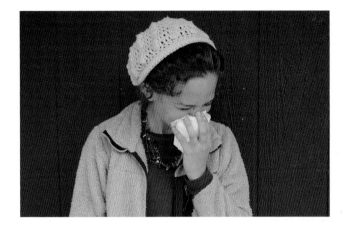

patient might need no more than a pad of gauze and a piece of tape, or the patient might be in cardiac arrest, and you are the one to respond. Often there is nothing you can do other than call 911, and you are the one to make the call—and that's great. Often knowing when to summon professional aid is the most life-saving act you can do. (Scattered throughout this book are "Red Lights," reminders of when to call for professional help if you haven't already.) All of these situations, small and big, require "first aid," and most of these situations are covered in this book.

Who knows when it all started? Evidence discovered in what remains of prehistoric people shows that broken bones were "set" and the bones healed appropriately. Undoubtedly, although unverifiable, some individuals must have shown particular though amateurish skill and/or interest in caring for the sick and injured, and to these ancient people we may, at least loosely, apply the label "first-aid provider."

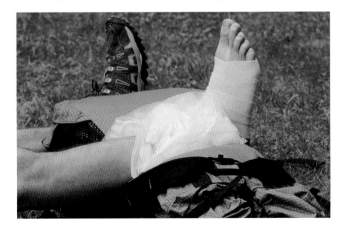

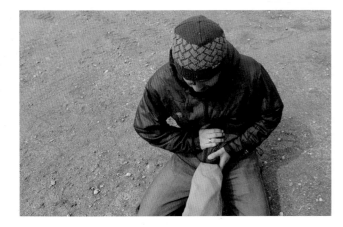

More fantastically, evidence of brain surgery, including the surgical implements, has been found dating back at least nine thousand years. There must have been some sort of "professional" training for those people opening human skulls for helpful reasons, so let's call these people the first "physicians." In some long-gone historic era, therefore, a difference between the lay provider and the professional provider became well established.

The earliest recorded provision of first aid was by religious knights of the eleventh century. The Order of St. John not only provided first aid but also trained other knights to take care of common injuries incurred in battle. Battlefields, and the need to provide care for the wounded, have been at the forefront of the development of first aid ever since. In the 1860s, a group of concerned people convened in Geneva, Switzerland, and gave birth to the Red Cross with the goal of aiding "sick and wounded soldiers in the field." The term "first aid," however, did not appear in print until 1878 when civilian ambulance services were formed to bring the "first" treatment to people in need as a form of national "aid."

About three years later, on May 21, 1881, the American Red Cross was founded by Clara Barton and a few friends in Washington, DC, and she was inspired by the first-aid movement that spread from Geneva and was already under way in other countries.

Whenever and wherever it started, and to whomever we give credit, the fact remains that you as a first-aid provider are part of a long and distinguished history. And that history is filled with kindness and compassion as well as skill.

The history of first aid is also filled with books about first aid, quite a few of them over the past thirty years written by me. What makes this book unique is approximately five hundred color photographs that not only help you learn what to do but also bring to life the process of caring for those in need of medical assistance. Even those with no interest in reading can learn something by just looking at the pictures. (I don't recommend just looking at the pictures. I am only pointing out that aspect of the book.)

And another aspect of this book, although not unique, is that it addresses a number of circumstances—let's call them "disaster situations"—where you may be cut off from rapid access to professional help via dialing 911 or jumping

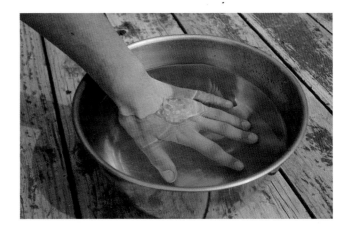

into the car for a short drive to the emergency room. For example, you would not typically choose to close a deep cut or attempt to put a dislocated shoulder back where it belongs. But if the roads are washed out, you might wish to know more about some injuries and illnesses than you'll find in a standard first-aid book.

Finally, to be completely honest, everything you need is not here. Sophocles, the Greek playwright, wrote, "Although you think you may know a thing, you have no certainty until you try." It's sort of like riding a bicycle. You can learn all about bicycle riding, but you can't do the thing until you get onto a bike and push off. You will learn a lot about CPR in this book, and you will "see" CPR being performed, but you need to take a CPR course to be sure you can do the thing. And the same may be said of many first-aid skills. So, if you really want to be the best first-aid provider possible, read this book *and* take a first-aid course.

OPEN THE AIRWAY

To assure you have a patient, you need to be assured of an airway

As a first-aid provider, fortunately you will find that most of your patients are able to breathe without any assistance from you. When they cannot, it is a situation immediately stressful and fearful for rescuer and patients alike. Take away the ability to breathe for only a few minutes, and the heart begins to weaken—and soon will stop beating. Few first-aid skills are as critically important as those involving a human's airway.

Conscious patients will speak, and you'll know they have an open airway. Make it a practice, however, to ask patients if breathing is a problem. Not all breathing difficulties are readily apparent. You will learn more about breathing difficulties later in this book.

When you are not sure if someone is breathing, ask, "Are you okay?" or a similar question. If you get no response, ask again in a much louder voice. If you still get no response, try to get a reaction to pain by rubbing your knuckles aggressively

Head-tilt/chin-lift

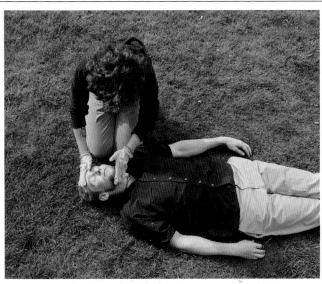

- Use the head-tilt/chin-lift to open the airway of an unresponsive patient.

- Press down firmly on the forehead of the patient, tilting the head back, while at the same time lifting the chin up until it is pointing "toward the sky."

- This movement lifts the tongue from the back of the throat to open the airway.

- It is more common for a rescuer to lift the chin too little rather than too much.

Opening the Mouth

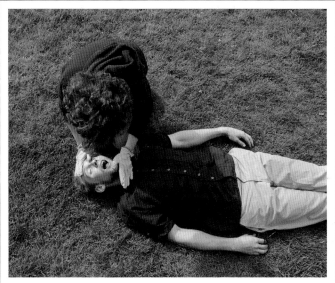

- You need to open the mouth of an unresponsive patient to check for obstructions (and later to listen for the sound of breathing).

- Keep pressure on the forehead to maintain the head-tilt/chin-lift.

- Open the mouth wide enough to allow visual inspection of the oral cavity.

- If you see a foreign body in the mouth, gently remove it. If you see nothing, do *not* blindly sweep the mouth with a finger.

against the sternum in the middle of the chest or pinching the back of an arm. With no response at all, you need to open the airway.

In most situations, you will want unresponsive patients on their back, a position that allows you to perform a head-tilt/chin-lift to open the airway.

ZOOM

Roll a patient as a unit, which means roll the head, shoulders, and trunk simultaneously, keeping the spine of the patient in line as much as possible.

Jaw-thrust

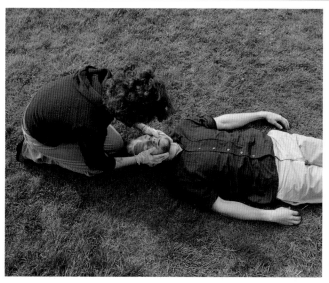

- Consider using the jaw-thrust to open the airway of an unresponsive patient when you suspect the patient's neck could have been damaged.

- Using both your hands, place your thumbs beside the patient's nose and your fingers along the line of the patient's jaw.

- Without tilting the patient's head, lift the jaw up. It does not need to lift much to open the airway.

- The jaw-thrust is seldom used by nonprofessionals— and the head-tilt/chin-lift may be used instead.

Opening the Airway

- Immediately open the airway of unresponsive patients.

- Use the head-tilt/chin-lift.

- Open the mouth and check for objects in the mouth.

- Remove any objects you can see.

CHECK FOR BREATHING

An airway is not enough unless the patient is using it to breathe

After performing a head-tilt/chin-lift on an unresponsive patient, remember to hold the mouth of the patient open and look inside. If you see any objects in the mouth—chewing gum, broken teeth, partially chewed food, and so forth—remove them quickly but gently from the mouth. If you see nothing, keep your fingers out of the patient's mouth.

To check for breathing, bend low enough over the patient to place your ear very near the patient's open mouth. Use the ear that allows you to look down the length of the patient's body. Look, listen, and feel for breathing. Look for movement of the chest. Listen for the sound of breathing. Feel for air movement against your ear and cheek. You can also use your hand that lifted the patient's chin to press lightly on the chest of the patient just below the sternum to feel for movement. Check for breathing for approximately ten seconds.

Check for breathing in a child (one to eight years of age) in

Check for Breathing

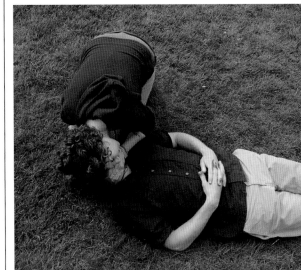

- Breathing is indicated by air moving in and out of the patient's chest. Look, listen, and feel for the movement of air.

- With the airway open, *look* for the rise and fall of the patient's chest.

- Place your ear near the patient's mouth and *listen* for the sound of air moving in and out.

- You may also be able to *feel* the patient's warm exhalation against your ear and cheek.

Check for Chest Movement

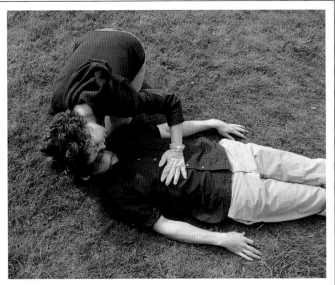

- With some patients, such as heavily clothed patients, you may feel chest movement without seeing it. Feeling movement also adds to your assurance that the patient is breathing.

- With one hand, press gently on the patient's chest just below the sternum (the breastbone). Be sure you are touching the upper abdominal area.

- You may feel more movement in the upper abdominal area than in the chest itself.

- Look, listen, and feel for breathing for ten seconds.

the same way you check in an adult. In an infant, however, perform the head-tilt/chin-lift only to the point where the head and chin are just past the midline of the body and in a neutral position, not extended back as in an adult and child.

Checking an Infant

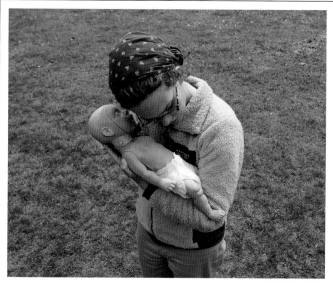

- Although it may seem obvious, remember to move an infant with more gentleness than you use with an adult.

- Use a head-tilt/chin-lift, but do *not* extend an infant's head back much past the neutral position.

- Look, listen, and feel for breathing as you do when checking an adult. And remember that infants normally breathe faster than an adult breathes.

- Once again, check for breathing for ten seconds.

Breathing Checklist

- Open the airway.

- Look, listen, and feel for breathing.

- Feel for movement of the chest and upper abdomen.

- Check for ten seconds.

ADULT AIRWAY CLEARING 1

A conscious adult may have an airway blocked with a foreign body

Sometimes a conscious person has a foreign body obstructing the airway. The most common foreign body is food. The object usually lodges near the opening to the windpipe (trachea), and the blockage may be partial or complete. With a complete blockage, the person cannot speak or cough—or breathe. This person requires immediate first aid.

With someone who appears to have a blocked airway, identify yourself as someone who can help and ask, "Are you choking?" If the response is a nod of affirmation, ask, "Can you speak?" If the response is negative, then:

Move to stand behind the person. Wrap your arms around the person about waist high and with your elbows out, away from the person. Make a fist and place it, thumb in, on the midline of the person's abdomen, just above the navel and well below the xiphoid process (the point of cartilage extending below the lower end of the sternum). Grab your

Step 1: Check for Choking

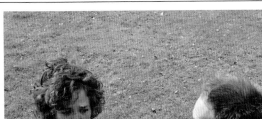

- Encourage the mildly choking, coughing patient to keep coughing, but do not interfere.

- If the patient goes silent or makes high-pitched, wheezing sounds attempting to breathe, identify yourself clearly as someone who can help.

- Do not immediately step behind the patient and out of sight of the patient. Maintain physical contact with the patient.

- Ask, "Are you choking?" People who can speak are mildly choking and do not require first aid.

Step 2: Position Yourself

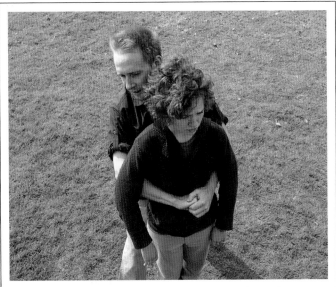

- Step behind the patient, and reach around to find the belly button. You may need to kneel behind a child.

- With both arms wrapped around the patient, make a fist with one hand and place it, thumb in, just above the belly button.

- Grasp your fist with your other hand.

- Lift your elbows up and out. You do not want to squeeze the patient with your arms, but, instead, press into the patient's abdomen with your fist.

fist with your other hand, and pull in and upward vigorously, a motion intended to expel the air from the patient's chest and the object from the airway. Repeat this abdominal thrust until the object is expelled or the person goes unconscious.

Note: With a choking pregnant woman, position your hands in the middle of the sternum instead of on the abdomen.

YELLOW LIGHT

When you clear the airway of a choking person using an abdominal thrust, that person is usually okay. But if the person complains of abdominal pain later, a doctor's evaluation is recommended.

Step 3: Abdominal Thrust

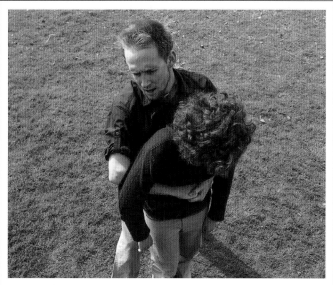

- Using both your arms simultaneously, pull sharply in and up.

- You must pull firmly enough to force the air out of the patient's chest, which will take the object blocking the airway with it.

- Continue performing abdominal thrusts until the patient's airway is open. When it is open, breathing will resume.

- If you do not clear the airway, the patient will pass out. With large patients, position yourself to control their body weight if they do.

Patient Loses Consciousness

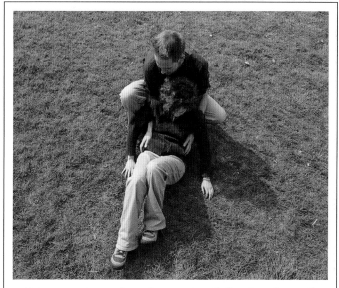

- If the airway is not cleared, the patient will lose consciousness and collapse in your arms. If your first attempts to clear the airway have failed, be prepared for this to happen.

- Tighten your arms, and step back to prevent the patient from falling face-first to the floor or ground.

- With as much control as possible, lower the patient to a face-up position.

- Immediately ask someone to call 911.

ADULT AIRWAY CLEARING 2

An unconscious adult may have an airway blocked with a foreign body

With an unconscious person who does not respond to any stimulus, ask someone to call 911, then open the airway, inspect for obstructions, and check for breathing—as explained earlier in this chapter. If you find no indication of breathing, seal your mouth over the patient's mouth (or use a rescue mask), and attempt to ventilate. If no air goes in, reposition the patient's

airway, and make a second attempt to ventilate. If air fails to go in on the second attempt (and the patient's chest does not rise), you may be dealing with a blocked airway.

Immediately start the chest compressions of CPR (see "Adult CPR"). The thirty compressions (at a rate of approximately one hundred per minute) will create enough pressure in the

Step 1: Check for an Airway

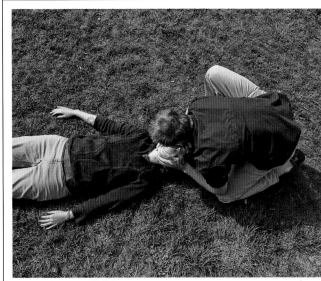

- When you find someone apparently unconscious, attempt to get a response by shouting and then by pinching the back of an arm.

- If you get no response, ask someone to call 911.

- Open the patient's airway with a head-tilt/chin-lift, check for and remove any obstructions visible in the mouth, and check for breathing.

- If you cannot detect breathing, attempt a rescue breath either via mouth-to-mouth or via a rescue mask.

Step 2: Reposition the Airway

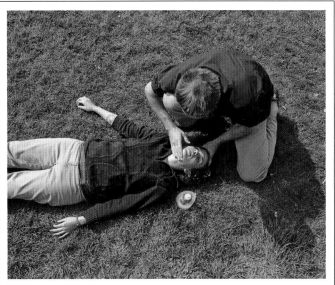

- If your attempt to breathe for the patient is unsuccessful on the first attempt, you may have failed to fully open the airway.

- Without fully opening the airway, the patient's tongue may be blocking your attempt at rescue breathing.

- Reposition the patient's airway with a second head-tilt/chin-lift, taking care to extend the head backward more than on the first attempt.

- Attempt a second rescue breath via mouth-to-mouth or via a rescue mask.

chest to force out a blockage.

After thirty compressions, open the airway, inspect inside the mouth for obstructions, and remove any that you see. If you remove a foreign body, or if you don't, attempt to ventilate again. If air fails to go in, reposition the airway and make a second attempt. If the second attempt fails, return to thirty more chest compressions. Repeat this process until the airway is cleared and you can either ventilate the patient (see "Rescue Breathing") or the patient begins to breathe without assistance.

Step 3: Clearing the Airway

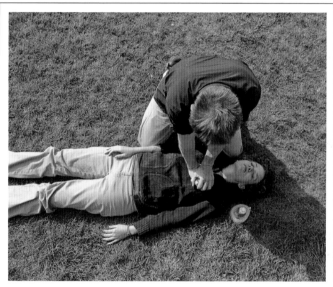

- If a second rescue breath fails to go in, the patient may have a foreign body airway obstruction.

- Perform thirty chest compressions as you do when performing CPR.

- Open the airway with a head-tilt/chin-lift, open the mouth and check for and remove visible objects, and attempt a rescue breath.

- If your breath fails to go in, reposition the patient's head and try again. If your second attempt fails, perform thirty compressions again—and repeat these steps until you clear the airway.

············ RED ● LIGHT ·············

Anyone who has choked long enough to pass out should be evaluated by a physician to make sure no serious internal damage has occurred.

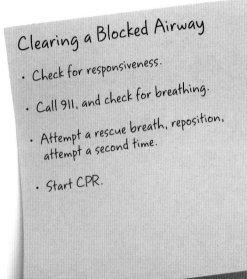

Clearing a Blocked Airway

- Check for responsiveness.

- Call 911, and check for breathing.

- Attempt a rescue breath, reposition, attempt a second time.

- Start CPR.

INFANT AIRWAY CLEARING

An infant's airway is not the same as an adult's airway

With an infant (under one year of age) who is coughing or gagging, respond as you would with an adult—do not interfere.

If the baby's attempts to breathe sound high-pitched, or if the baby goes silent or grows too weak to cough, hold the baby while opening the airway. Do not extend the baby's head back, but keep it in neutral alignment with the body. Inspect the airway, and remove any obstructions you can see.

If the baby is still choking, sandwich the baby between your forearms, supporting the head, and turn the baby face down with the head lower than the body. Deliver five back blows with the heel of your hand, between the baby's shoulder blades. If your forearm beneath the baby is placed against your thigh, your back blows will be more effective.

After five back blows, while still supporting the baby's head, turn the baby face up. Place two of your fingers on the

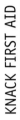

Step 1: Check for an Airway

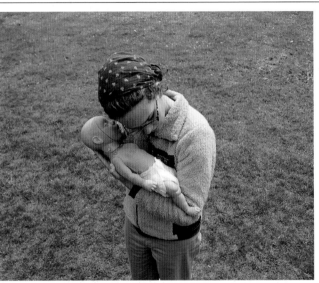

- Hold the baby on one arm with the head held securely and in line with the baby's body.

- Open the mouth wide enough to allow visible inspection. If you see an object in the mouth, remove it, but do not

- blindly sweep your finger through the baby's mouth.

- Attempt to breathe in a rescue "puff" of air.

- If your rescue breath fails to go in, tilt the baby's head back a little, and attempt a second rescue breath.

Step 2: Back Blows

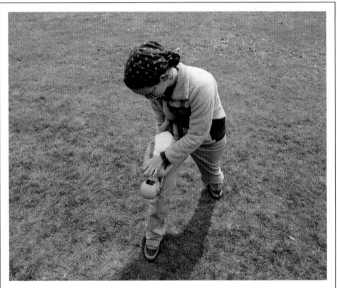

- If your second attempt at rescue breathing fails, the baby may have a foreign body airway obstruction.

- With the head held securely, "sandwich" the baby between your arms, and turn the baby face down with the head lower than the body.

- Lower the arm supporting the baby until it is supported by your thigh.

- With the heel of your hand, deliver five back blows between the baby's shoulder blades.

middle of the chest just below nipple line and compress the chest five times. Compress about one-third the thickness of the chest.

Repeat the back blows and chest compressions until the airway is cleared, until the baby starts to cry or cough, or until the baby goes unconscious.

If the baby goes unconscious with a blocked airway, start CPR (see "Infant CPR").

···· RED ● LIGHT ····

Any infant who has had a blocked airway long enough to cause unconsciousness should be evaluated by a physician as soon as possible.

Step 3: Chest Thrusts

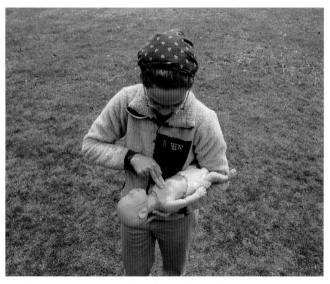

- While still supporting the head, turn the baby face up, and support arm and baby once again on your thigh.

- Place two fingers on the middle of the baby's chest just below nipple line. Push down about one-third the depth of the chest. Push down five times.

- Check the mouth, removing any visible objects.

- Repeat these steps until the baby starts to breathe, cry, or cough.

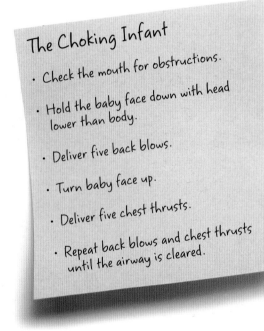

The Choking Infant

- Check the mouth for obstructions.

- Hold the baby face down with head lower than body.

- Deliver five back blows.

- Turn baby face up.

- Deliver five chest thrusts.

- Repeat back blows and chest thrusts until the airway is cleared.

RESCUE BREATHING

When someone is not breathing, you may have to breathe for that person

The air you inhale contains about 21 percent oxygen. The air you exhale contains about 16 percent, so you can breathe for someone who is not breathing by exhaling into that person.

After sending someone to call 911, and after you have opened the airway and determined that an unresponsive person is not breathing (see "Check for Breathing"), use the thumb and forefinger of your hand holding the patient's forehead to pinch closed the nostrils. If the nose is not pinched, the air you breathe in will escape through the nose. Hold the patient's mouth open with your other hand, open your mouth wide, and seal it over the patient's mouth. If you are using a rescue mask, it may fit over the nose and mouth,

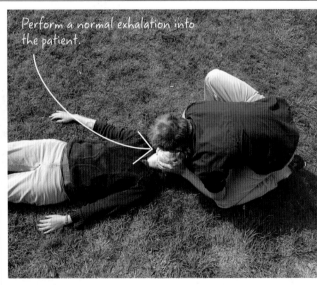

Breathing for an Adult

Perform a normal exhalation into the patient.

- A patient who is not breathing but who has a heart-beat needs someone to breathe for him or her.

- Hold the airway open with a head-tilt/chin-lift, pinch the nostrils shut, and take a normal breath. Seal your mouth over the patient's mouth and exhale normally.

- You may use a rescue mask instead of mouth-to-mouth.

- A rescue breath should last only one second, with enough volume to make the chest rise.

- Deliver ten to twelve rescue breaths per minute.

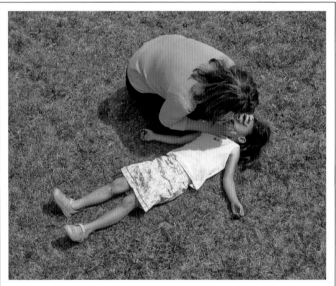

Breathing for a Child

- Rescue breathing for a child is the same as for an adult.

- Hold the airway open with a head-tilt/chin-lift, pinch the nostrils shut, and take a normal breath. Seal your mouth over the patient's mouth and exhale normally. You may use a rescue mask instead of mouth-to-mouth.

- A rescue breath should last only one second, with enough volume to make the chest rise. Small children will require a smaller rescue breath.

- Deliver ten to twelve rescue breaths per minute.

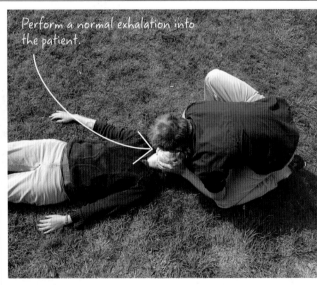

KNACK FIRST AID

and you don't have to pinch the nose shut. Deliver two slow breaths, about one second each, waiting a moment between breaths for the air to escape the patient's lungs. The patient's chest will rise and fall, indicating the air has gone in and out. Your inhalations and exhalations should be normal, not exaggerated.

If air does not go in, reposition the airway, and attempt to ventilate again. If your second attempt fails, you probably have a patient with a blocked airway (see "Adult Airway Clearing 2").

Once you have delivered two breaths to the patient, check for signs of circulation (see "Adult CPR").

With a patient who has signs of circulation but who is not breathing, continue mouth-to-mouth (or mouth-to-mask) rescue breathing until spontaneous breathing returns and/ or help arrives. Deliver ten to twelve rescue breaths per minute, or one rescue breath every five or six seconds.

Note: Patients with a stoma, a permanent opening surgically implanted in the trachea, should have rescue breaths delivered through the stoma.

Breathing for an Infant

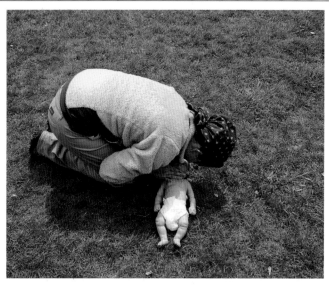

- Perform a head-tilt/chin-lift to open the baby's airway, but do not hyperextend the head as you do with adults and children.

- Take a normal breath, and seal your mouth over the baby's mouth and nose.

- Breathe in gently, just a puff of air, enough to make the chest rise. Each breath should last about one second.

- Breathe for an infant at a rate of one breath every three to five seconds.

Rescue Breathing

- Open the airway with a head-tilt/chin-lift.

- Pinch the nostrils shut with adults and children.

- Seal your mouth over the patient's mouth (or mouth and nose for an infant).

- Exhale normally, enough to make the chest rise.

- Each rescue breath should take one second.

ADULT CPR

Quick action gives a breathless, pulseless victim the best chance of life

Cardiac arrest, the cessation of useful heart muscle activity, marks the moment of clinical death in a human. Between the moment of cardiac arrest and the cessation of brain activity (biological death), there is a window of opportunity to apply the skills of cardiopulmonary resuscitation (CPR) and, perhaps, save the victim.

As soon as you realize you have an unresponsive patient, activate the emergency response system—call 911 or send someone to call 911. Then open and quickly inspect the airway (see "Open the Airway"). Then look, listen, and feel for breathing for approximately ten seconds (see "Check for Breathing"). If you find no indication of breathing, perform

Step 1: Check for Breathing

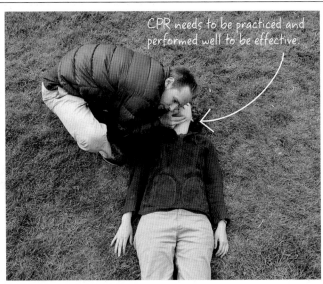

CPR needs to be practiced and performed well to be effective.

- Remember: The first phase of CPR is determining if the patient is responsive. If you get no response from the patient, go call 911, or, even better, send someone to call 911.

- Then position the patient flat, face up, on a firm surface.

- Perform a head-tilt/chin-lift, open the patient's mouth, look inside, and remove any visible obstructions.

- Place your ear near the patient's mouth while looking down the length of the patient.

Step 2: Rescue Breathing

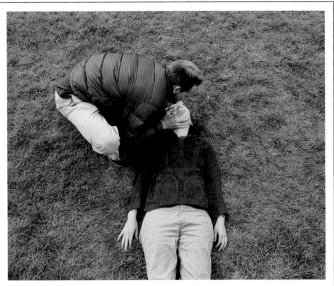

- If you can detect no breathing after ten seconds of looking, listening, and feeling for breathing, pinch the nostrils shut, and seal your mouth over the patient's mouth, or use your rescue mask, and give a rescue breath.

- Your rescue breath should be a normal exhalation, about one second long.

- If your first breath goes in, immediately give a second breath.

- If your first breath does not go in, reposition the patient's head, and give two breaths.

two slow artificial ventilations (see "Rescue Breathing").

Check for circulation, which in this case means a pulse. Place two or three of your fingers gently on the "Adam's apple" (larynx), and slide your fingers off into the "valley" between the larynx and the large neck muscle. At the same time, look down the length of the body, checking for other signs of circulation, which include breathing, coughing, or moving.

With no signs of circulation, begin CPR. CPR is performed at a 30:2 ratio—thirty chest compressions to two rescue breaths.

CPR

Step 3: Check for Circulation

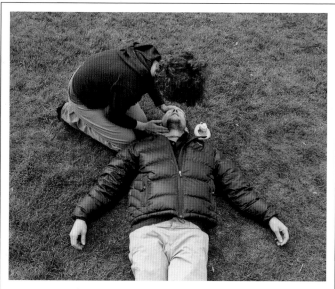

- After two rescue breaths, look down the length of the patient to check for signs of circulation (heart activity).

- Coughing, breathing, and/or any moving are signs of heart activity.

- You may also use two or three fingers to check for a pulse at the neck.

- Place your fingers gently on the patient's Adam's apple, and slide off into the space between the Adam's apple and the neck muscle to check for a pulse. Check for ten seconds.

Step 4: Chest Compressions

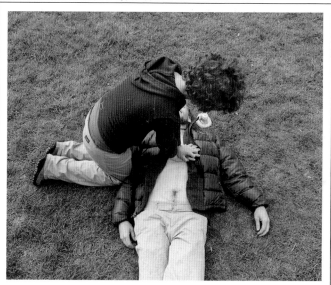

- If no circulation is found, bare the patient's chest, and place the heel of one hand on the middle of the sternum.

- Place your second hand over your first, and straighten and lock your elbows.

- Lean forward in order to press straight down, and perform thirty compressions at a rate of one hundred per minute.

- After each thirty compressions, give another two breaths, and repeat 30:2 five times before checking for circulation. If no circulation, keep up the cycle of 30:2.

ADULT A.E.D.

An automated external defibrillator gives the victim a better chance than CPR alone

Ventricular fibrillation is rapid, quivering, incomplete contractions of the muscle fibers of the ventricles of the heart, the result most often of a heart attack. The patient is in cardiac arrest, without detectable breathing or heartbeat. A defibrillator stops fibrillation by stopping heart activity via an electrical shock. If it is applied soon enough, the heart may start again under its own electrical impulse and in a normal and useful rhythm. An automated external defibrillator (A.E.D.) decides if a shock is advised and prepares for delivery of the shock if it is placed correctly on the patient. Use of an A.E.D., far more than CPR alone, greatly increases the chance that the patient will survive.

CPR

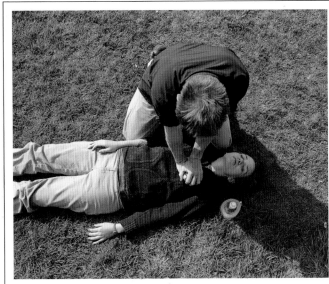

Pads

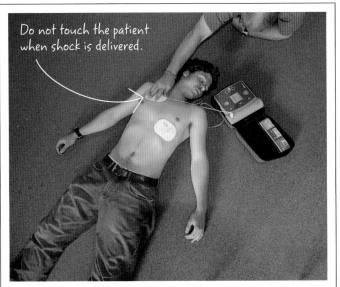

Do not touch the patient when shock is delivered.

- A patient in cardiac arrest has the best chance of survival if CPR is started immediately.

- An automated external defibrillator (A.E.D.) assumes that CPR has been started. Always start CPR and send someone to get an A.E.D. if one is nearby.

- If the A.E.D. arrives with someone who cannot use it, ask that person to take over chest compressions while you operate the A.E.D.

- Interrupt CPR as little as possible while setting up the machine.

- An A.E.D. has two pads that must be connected to cables, and the cables must be plugged into the machine. The A.E.D. may arrive with the pads connected.

- The adhesive sides of the pads must be attached to bare skin.

- The pads will have illustrations telling you where to put them. If you see no illustrations, then one pad goes above the right nipple, and the other one goes on the side below the left nipple.

An A.E.D. assumes that CPR will be started on the patient while someone else brings the A.E.D. If you are alone, you may choose to perform five cycles (about two minutes) of CPR before using the A.E.D. Once the A.E.D. is turned on, you will hear directions about how to proceed—and you should follow those directions.

The A.E.D.'s two pads are sticky, and they must be placed on the skin of the patient's chest wall, one below the right shoulder and the other below the left nipple. Most pads have illustrations on them showing where to place them.

The patient should not be touched or moved while the A.E.D. is analyzing—and the device will remind you of this. If it decides to deliver a shock, it will tell you when to push the "shock" button.

After the shock is delivered, CPR should be immediately resumed. Two minutes later, the A.E.D. will ask you to stop CPR while it decides if another shock is to be delivered.

The Shock

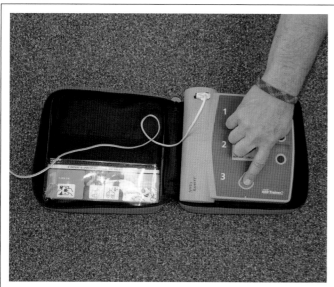

- When the A.E.D. is turned on, it will tell you to place the pads if you haven't done so already.

- Stop CPR, and move back. No one can be touching the patient while the A.E.D. works.

- The A.E.D. will analyze the patient's heart, and the A.E.D. will tell you when to push the shock button.

- After the shock, the A.E.D. will tell you to resume CPR if needed. Leave the pads in place and the machine on. It will soon reanalyze.

Using an A.E.D.

- Start CPR.

- Plug in the pads, and place the pads on bare skin.

- Turn on the machine if you haven't yet.

- Move back.

- Push the shock button when told to by the A.E.D.

- Resume CPR if told to by the A.E.D.

CHILD CPR

A few differences distinguish child CPR from adult CPR

Cardiac arrest in a child (about one to eight years of age) is rarely the result of heart disease. Usually the cause is a lack of sufficient oxygen from suffocation, injury, or an illness. For that reason, if you're alone you should give two minutes of CPR immediately before phoning 911.

Open the airway, and deliver rescue breaths to a child the same as you would for an adult. With a small child, however, moderate your artificial ventilations. Small lungs simply need less air to fill them than large lungs. The volume should be just enough to make the chest rise.

Check for a pulse and other signs of circulation the same as you would for an adult. Chest compressions are performed as on an adult: thirty compressions (performed rhythmically to a depth of approximately one-third the thickness of the patient's chest) to every two rescue breaths.

If two rescuers are available to do CPR on a child, the ratio

Step 1: Check for Breathing

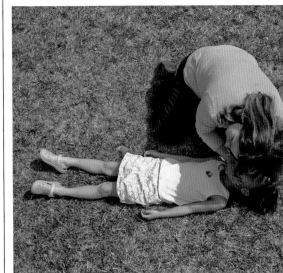

- With a patient between the ages of one and eight years, CPR is almost the same as for an adult. If you get no response from the patient, start CPR immediately.

- Send someone to call 911, or go make the call yourself *after* two minutes (five cycles) of CPR.

- Perform a head-tilt/chin-lift, open the patient's mouth, look inside, and remove any visible obstructions.

- Place your ear near the patient's mouth while looking down the length of the patient.

Step 2: Rescue Breathing

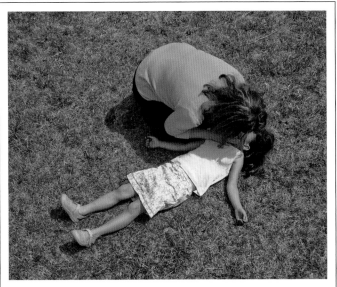

- If you can detect no breathing after ten seconds of looking, listening, and feeling for breathing, pinch the nostrils shut, seal your mouth over the patient's mouth, and give a rescue breath.

- Your rescue breath should be a normal exhalation, about one second long.

- If your first breath goes in, immediately give a second breath.

- If your first breath does not go in, you probably failed to open the airway enough. Reposition the patient's head, and give two breaths.

should be changed to fifteen chest compressions for every two ventilations.

With a child who is unconscious and bluish in color but who has a pulse, count the heartbeats for fifteen seconds and multiply by four. If the child's pulse is less than sixty beats per minute, consider starting CPR. This child is not circulating oxygenated blood quickly enough.

CPR

Step 3: Check for Circulation

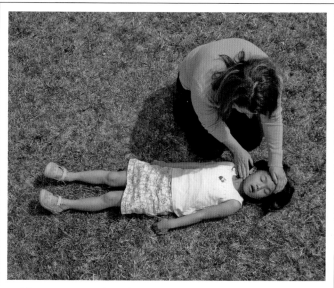

- After two rescue breaths, look down the length of the patient to check for signs of circulation (heart activity).

- Coughing, breathing, and/or any moving are signs of heart activity.

- You may also use two or three fingers to check for a pulse at the neck.

- Place your fingers gently on the patient's Adam's apple, and slide off into the space between the Adam's apple and the neck muscle to check for a pulse. Check for ten seconds.

Step 4: Chest Compressions

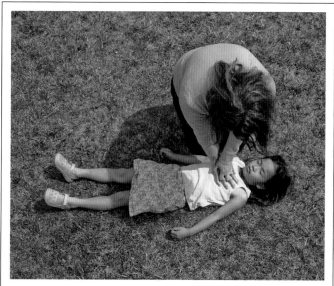

- If no circulation is found, bare the chest, and place the heel of one hand on the middle of the sternum.

- With a small child, you may need to use only one hand.

- Perform thirty compressions at a rate of one hundred per minute. Press down about one-third the depth of the chest.

- After thirty compressions, give another two breaths, and repeat the cycle five times before checking for a return of circulation. If no circulation is detected, continue with CPR.

CHILD A.E.D.

An automated external defibrillator for a child is not exactly the same as an adult's

Use of an automated external defibrillator (A.E.D.) is recommended for children in cardiac arrest. A child may be defined as someone between about one year of age and about eight years of age or up to about fifty-five pounds in weight. As with adults, the use of an A.E.D. on a child greatly increases the chance of a favorable outcome as opposed to use of CPR alone.

Many A.E.D.s—but not all—are now equipped to deliver smaller doses of electricity through either smaller pads (child pads) or another means to reduce the energy dose.

The procedure for using an A.E.D. on a child is exactly the same as on an adult (see "Adult A.E.D."). CPR should be started immediately. If you're alone, give CPR for two minutes before

CPR

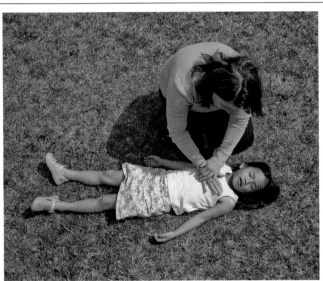

- A child in cardiac arrest has the best chance of survival if CPR is started immediately.

- An automated external defibrillator (A.E.D.) assumes that CPR has been started. Always start CPR, and send someone to get an A.E.D. if one is nearby.

- If the A.E.D. arrives with someone who cannot use it, ask that person to take over chest compressions while you operate the A.E.D.

- Interrupt CPR as little as possible while setting up the machine.

A.E.D.

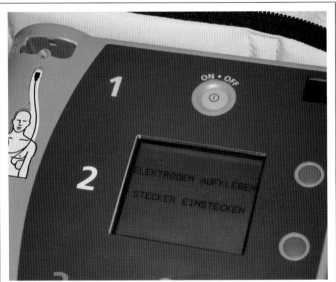

- A child A.E.D. delivers a smaller shock via either smaller pads or a way to reduce the electrical charge.

- As with an adult A.E.D., the adhesive sides of the pads must be attached to bare skin.

- The pads will have illustrations telling you where to put them. If you see no illustrations, one pad goes above the right nipple, and the other one goes on the side below the left nipple.

calling for help and/or while the A.E.D. is being brought, turned on, and attached to the child. The pads, as on an adult, are placed on bare skin, one just below the right shoulder and the other just below the left nipple. As with an adult, you should follow the audible directions supplied by the A.E.D.

CPR

The Shock

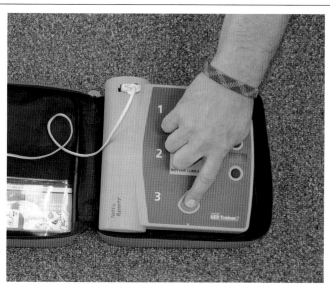

- When the A.E.D. is turned on, it will tell you to place the pads if you haven't done so already.

- Stop CPR, and move back. No one can be touching the patient while the A.E.D. works.

- The A.E.D. will analyze the child's heart, and the A.E.D. will tell you when to push the shock button.

- After the shock, the A.E.D. will tell you to resume CPR if needed. Leave the pads in place and the machine on. It will soon reanalyze.

Use of Child A.E.D.

- Start CPR.

- Plug in the pads, and place the pads on bare skin.

- Turn on the machine if you haven't yet.

- Move back.

- Push the shock button when told to by the A.E.D.

- Resume CPR if told to by the A.E.D.

INFANT CPR 1

During the first year, a baby requires a different approach to CPR

To be effective—and it can be effective—CPR on an infant (someone in the first year of life) is not the same as CPR on an adult.

To check for responsiveness in an infant, tap the bottom of the foot, and speak in a loud voice. Say something like, "Are you alright?" If the baby does not respond, send someone to call 911.

Open the airway with a head-tilt/chin-lift, but do not extend the baby's head much past a neutral position. Extension much past neutral may shut off the short airway of an infant.

Holding the head in line, place your ear near the mouth, and look down the baby's body, looking, listening, and feeling for breathing. Check for breathing for about ten seconds. If you see no indication of breathing, seal your mouth over the baby's nose and mouth, and give two small, gentle breaths, about one second per breath. Your rescue breaths

Step 1: Check for Responsiveness

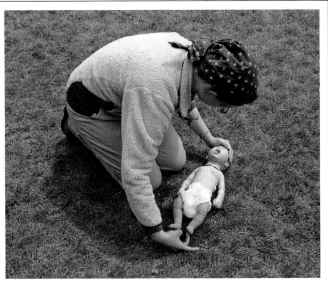

- Call out loudly in an attempt to get a response from the infant.

- With no response to a verbal stimulus, flick the infant's foot or tap the infant on the shoulder.

- If the infant is unresponsive, send someone to call 911, and continue to follow the steps that follow.

- If you are alone, you should delay calling 911. Continue to follow the steps that follow, and go call 911 after two minutes of CPR.

Step 2: Open the Airway

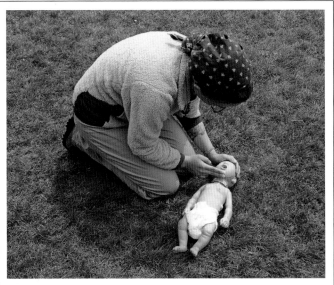

- Quickly but gently place the infant face up on a firm surface.

- Perform a head-tilt/chin-lift, but do *not* tilt the infant's head back much past neutral. The little airway will be open in the neutral or just past the neutral position.

- Gently open the infant's mouth, and check for visible obstructions.

- Remove anything visible in the infant's mouth, but otherwise do not stick a finger into the mouth.

should be just enough to make the chest rise. Pause briefly between breaths to allow the chest to relax.

If your breaths do not go in, reposition the baby's head, and try again. You may have tilted the head back too far. If your breaths still will not go in, the baby's airway may be blocked, requiring airway clearing (see "Infant Airway Clearing").

Step 3: Check for Breathing

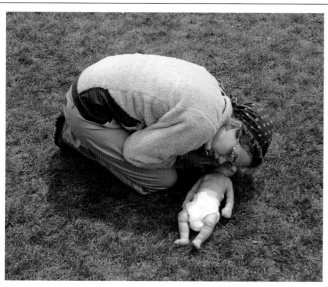

- With the mouth held open, place your ear against the infant's mouth while looking down the length of the infant's body.

- Look for the rise and fall of the chest that tell you that the baby is breathing. Other movement may also be a sign that the baby is breathing.

- You may be able to feel the baby's breath against your cheek or hear the sound of the baby breathing.

- Check for breathing for no more than ten seconds.

Step 4: Rescue Breathing

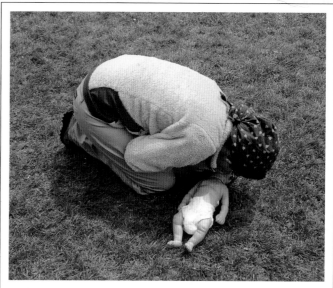

- If the infant is not breathing, seal your mouth over the baby's nose and mouth, and give two gentle puffs of rescue air.

- Remember that a baby's lungs are tiny and that too much air can damage the lungs and fill the baby's stomach with air.

- Your breaths should be just enough to make the small chest rise.

- Each breath should take no more than one second. Pause briefly between the two breaths.

INFANT CPR 2
Babies require different care because they are not little adults

Once you have determined that the infant is unresponsive and not breathing (see "Infant CPR 1"), you need to check for a heartbeat. The best place to check for a pulse on an infant is on the brachial artery, inside the upper arm. Check for about ten seconds.

In the absence of a pulse and prior to chest compressions, the baby needs to be placed on a flat, firm surface with the head not higher than the rest of the body. Bare the baby's chest, and place two fingers on the breastbone at the nipple line. Compress the chest about one-third the depth of the baby's body, and compress thirty times at a rate of about one hundred compressions per minute. (At this rate, it should take you less than twenty-three seconds to do the thirty compressions.)

After thirty compressions, deliver two rescue breaths of about one second each, allowing the chest to deflate in between.

Check for Circulation

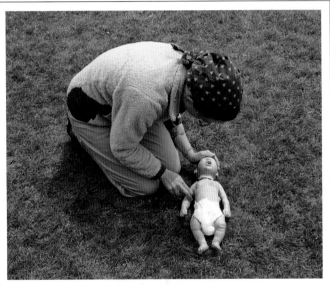

- After two rescue puffs of air, check for signs of circulation, signs that the infant's heart is beating.

- These signs may include breathing, coughing, or any moving, and you can check by observing the baby's body.

- You can check for a pulse by placing two of your fingers on the inside of the infant's upper arm not far below the armpit.

- Check for signs of circulation for ten seconds.

Compression Site

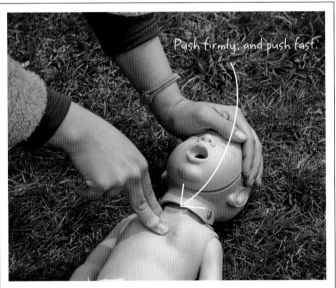

Push firmly, and push fast.

- In the absence of signs of circulation, you need to find the appropriate site to perform chest compressions.

- You must first bare the infant's chest. You cannot maintain contact with the appropriate site through clothing.

- Place the pads of two or three of your fingers on the center of the baby's sternum on an imaginary line between the nipples.

- Lift your hand so that your compressions will be straight down.

Continue to perform CPR at 30:2 until help arrives. If you are alone, perform five cycles of 30:2, or about two minutes of CPR, before going to call 911.

CPR

Chest Compressions

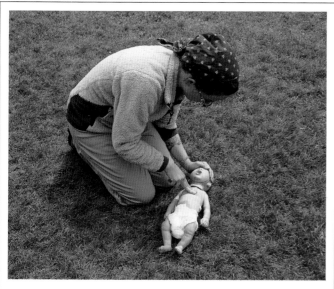

- Compress the chest about one-third the width of the chest.

- Push quickly and firmly and smoothly, not jerkily.

- Compress the chest thirty times at a rate of one hundred compressions per minute.

- After thirty compressions, give two more rescue puffs of air. Repeat the cycle for five times, or for approximately two minutes, and then check for a return of signs of circulation. If needed, continue the cycle of 30:2 until help arrives.

Infant CPR

- Check for responsiveness.

- Place the infant on a firm surface.

- Check for breathing. If none is detected, give two small rescue breaths.

- Check for circulation. If none is detected, perform thirty chest compressions.

- Continue the cycle of 30:2 as long as needed.

CHECK FOR BLEEDING

Life-threatening blood loss may not be immediately apparent

With every patient you provide first aid for, you need to know early whether that person is bleeding—and, more importantly, whether that person is seriously bleeding.

Conscious patients can often tell you if they're bleeding: They know if they are. Develop the first-aid habit of asking all patients, "Are you bleeding?" You also need to take a look at the wound or wounds and quickly decide if you need to take steps to stop the blood loss (see "Stop Bleeding").

But conscious patients will sometimes be distracted by their accident and/or by pain from other injuries and fail to be aware that they are bleeding. Therefore, incorporate into your approach to all patients a quick visual scan to check for bleeding.

With unconscious patients you need to do a blood sweep, a quick, hands-on check for bleeding in addition to a visual scan, remembering that wounds may lie hidden under bulky

Blood Sweep 1

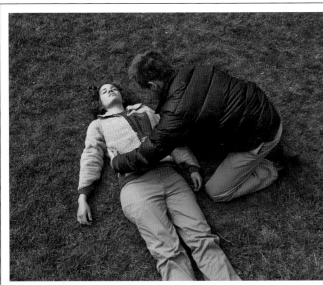

- The average adult male body contains between five and six liters of blood. The smaller the individual, the lower the blood volume.

- A one hundred-pound adolescent contains about three liters of blood, and a newborn about one-half liter.

- Ask conscious patients if they're bleeding, and quickly sweep the body of patients to check for blood loss.

- Be sure to check the hidden areas: underneath the patient and underneath clothing that could hide blood loss.

Blood Sweep 2

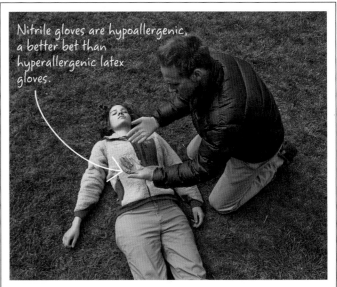

Nitrile gloves are hypoallergenic, a better bet than hyperallergenic latex gloves.

- Patients can bleed out into sand, rocks, a dense layer of leaves, and snow, leaving almost no trace on the surface upon which they are lying.

- Patients can bleed out into thick clothing and into water-resistant clothing, such as rainwear, without a visible trace on the surface of the clothing.

- These are the places into which you must stick your gloved hands.

- Take a look at your hands often while performing a blood sweep.

clothing or on the side of the patient hidden against the floor or ground. It is best to perform a blood sweep with gloved hands, and then check your gloves for blood.

Check the Wound

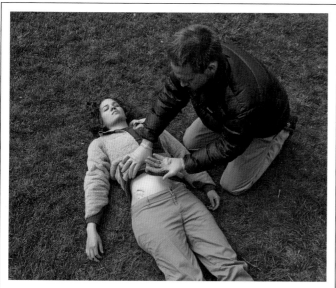

- Blood may also soak through clothing and appear on the surface of clothing.

- This blood may or may not be associated with a hole or tear in the clothing.

- It is in the best interest of the patient if you assume that any wet spot on clothing is blood until proven otherwise.

- Clothing must be removed from a wound, or the possibility of a wound, to reveal the wound at skin level.

The Blood Sweep

- Life-threatening blood loss can occur in minutes.

- Ask conscious patients if they are bleeding.

- Perform a visual scan of all patients.

- Perform a hands-on blood sweep of unconscious patients.

- Reveal all wounds at skin level.

BLEEDING & SHOCK

STOP BLEEDING 1
Serious blood loss must be stopped immediately

Serious blood loss from a wound must be stopped immediately. The most serious bleeding is arterial, rushing from an opening in an artery, rapidly leaving the patient, often spurting each time the patient's heart beats. Serious venous bleeding is coming from a large vein, flowing steadily from the patient. Serious blood loss often forms a fairly large pool of blood fairly quickly.

Fortunately, most bleeding can be stopped with pressure from your hand pressed directly over the wound. Large wounds may require you to pack the wound first with sterile gauze, although you can use any clean cloth in an emergency. Packing a wound allows you to apply direct pressure over a larger area. When the gauze or cloth is soaked with blood, it is best to apply a second layer of gauze or cloth and continue the pressure instead of removing the blood-soaked dressing.

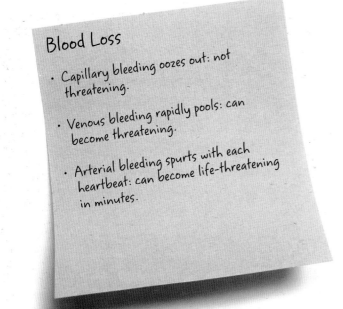

Blood Loss

- Capillary bleeding oozes out: not threatening.

- Venous bleeding rapidly pools: can become threatening.

- Arterial bleeding spurts with each heartbeat: can become life-threatening in minutes.

Direct Pressure

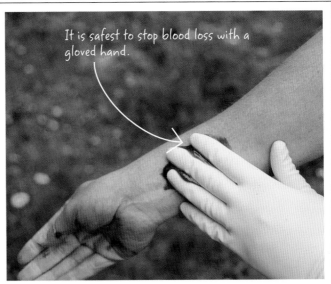

It is safest to stop blood loss with a gloved hand.

- Pressure from your hand or hands applied directly on the wound will stop most blood loss.

- It is better if there is absorbent material between your hands and the wound, but, if speed matters, you can use only your hands.

- You must press firmly enough to stop blood from leaving the patient's body.

- You may need to apply direct pressure for a long time before blood clots, allowing you to stop the pressure.

It is impossible to say how long you will have to apply direct pressure. Several variables are involved, including the size of the tear, whether the blood is coming from an artery, and how fast the patient's blood clots.

Packing a Wound

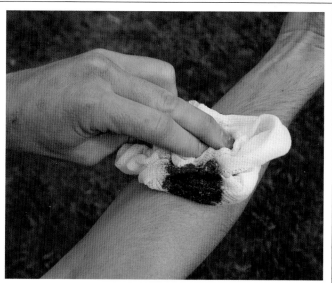

- Wounds larger than you can cover with your hands may resist direct pressure.

- Wounds that penetrate to deep within the patient's body may also resist direct pressure.

- In these cases, you need to pack absorbent material, preferably sterile gauze, into the wound prior to direct pressure. Do not be afraid to stuff the material aggressively into the wound.

- The bulky material will distribute your pressure and allow it to work.

Pressure Bandage

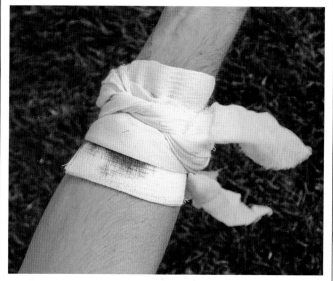

- A pressure bandage can be used when the blood loss is not life-threatening.

- This can be especially useful if you have other wounds or other patients to deal with.

- Press clean material, preferably sterile gauze, onto the wound. The material should be 1 inch thick or more.

- Hold pressure on the material with an elastic wrap or a band of any material you can tie around the body part. Pressure bandages must not be so tight that they cut off circulation.

BLEEDING & SHOCK

STOP BLEEDING 2
If direct pressure does not stop bleeding, consider a tourniquet

Although they are rare, you may encounter wounds that require a tourniquet to stop blood loss. A tourniquet is a band tied tightly enough around an arm or leg to stop all blood from passing the band. To ensure the best outcome for the patient, tourniquets need to be applied correctly.

Use material that you can fold into a wide band. The band should be about 4 inches wide. A narrow band, such as a rope, can cause localized damage to human tissue in minutes. A

large bandanna will also work well in a pinch.

Tie the band around the arm or leg just above the wound, "above" meaning on the side from which blood is flowing to the wound. Tie it tightly with an overhand knot. Then tie a stick, or anything rigid, into the band with a second overhand knot. Turn the stick until blood stops flowing from the wound—and then stop turning. If the tails of the material you used for the band are long enough, you can use them

Step 1: A Wide Band

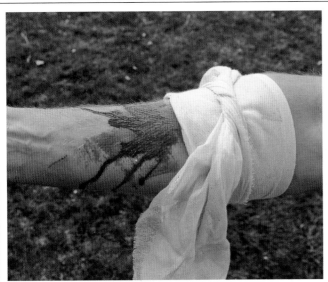

- Other than on battlefields, tourniquets are rarely needed, but when blood is being lost tremendously fast, a tourniquet can be life-saving.

- For the best results, use material that is wide—about 4 inches wide or more—and soft.

- Tie it around the arm or leg just above the wound, between the wound and the patient's heart.

- Use a simple overhand knot to tie the tourniquet, and pull it tight.

Step 2: Something Rigid

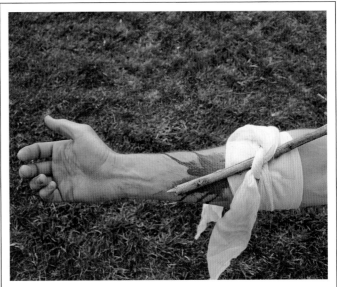

- You cannot apply a tourniquet without the use of something rigid with which you twist the material tied around the limb.

- It does not need to be long, but it does need to be strong, and it needs to be narrow.

- Place the rigid object on the overhand knot, and tie it in place with a second overhand knot.

- Twist the rigid object, tightening the wide band of material until all bleeding stops.

to tie the stick in place. If they are not long enough, you will have to find another piece of material to use.

················· RED ● LIGHT ··············

Even a properly applied tourniquet shuts off blood flow from the tourniquet to the rest of the arm or leg—so get to a hospital as soon as possible.

Step 3: Check for Pulse

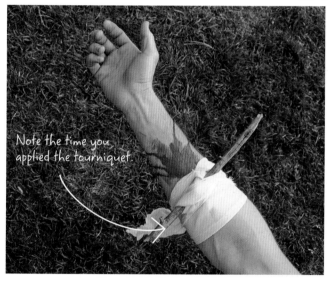

Note the time you applied the tourniquet.

- After bleeding stops, check for a pulse at the wrist or ankle. If you can find a pulse, the tourniquet is not tight enough. Tighten it more.

- A tourniquet that is too loose allows some arterial blood past but stops venous blood from returning.

- The limb will swell, and the swelling may increase the chance of irreversible harm.

- Once the tourniquet is tight enough, use the tails of the wide material to tie the rigid object in place.

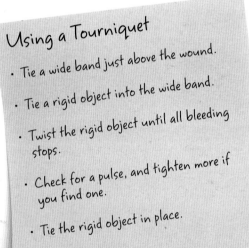

Using a Tourniquet

- Tie a wide band just above the wound.

- Tie a rigid object into the wide band.

- Twist the rigid object until all bleeding stops.

- Check for a pulse, and tighten more if you find one.

- Tie the rigid object in place.

- Note the time.

BLEEDING & SHOCK

29

SHOCK

Shock can have many causes with basically the same signs and symptoms

Perfusion is the constant bathing of the cells of a human body with life-sustaining blood under adequate pressure, the job of the cardiovascular system. Shock, whatever the cause, is inadequate perfusion. When vital organs receive inadequate perfusion, they are at risk of dying.

Inadequate perfusion can have many causes, including

failure of the heart to pump adequately after a heart attack; loss of blood, dehydration, and extensive burns, all reducing the fluid volume in the body; damage to the spinal cord that causes loss of adequate pressure within blood vessels; and a severe allergic reaction that can be a combination of shifting body fluid and loss of vascular tension.

Hypovolemic Shock

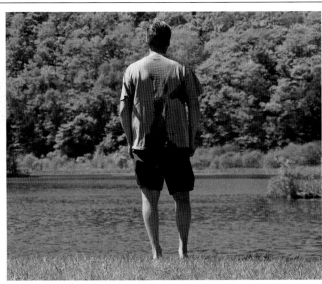

- Hypovolemic (or low-volume) shock results when loss of fluid volume from the body reaches the point where perfusion cannot be maintained.

- It can be caused by fluid lost in large amounts of sweat.

- It can be caused by profuse bleeding and by serious cases of diarrhea or vomiting, especially if both diarrhea *and* vomiting are involved.

- It can be caused by extensive burns due to the fact that fluid leaves the body from badly burned areas.

Cardiogenic Shock

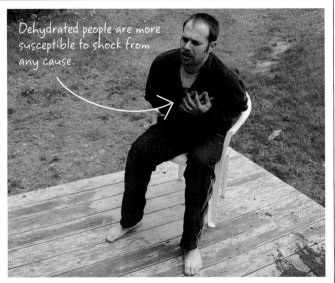

Dehydrated people are more susceptible to shock from any cause.

- Cardiogenic (heart-related) shock results when the heart cannot pump adequately enough to circulate blood well enough to maintain perfusion.

- The most common cause is a heart attack and the resulting death of a part of the heart.

- It could also be caused by severe irregularities in heart rhythm, problems related to the function of the heart muscle, and problems with the function of heart valves.

- Cardiogenic shock may come on devastatingly quickly.

Shock is progressive; the patient goes through stages because the body fights to compensate for the injury or illness. Patients can and often do worsen over time if inadequately treated.

Look for a patient who is increasingly anxious and confused. The heartbeat will speed up and weaken, and the breathing will quicken and become increasingly shallow as shock grows progressively worse. Look for pale, cool, clammy skin. The patient often grows weak, thirsty, and nauseous.

Vasogenic Shock

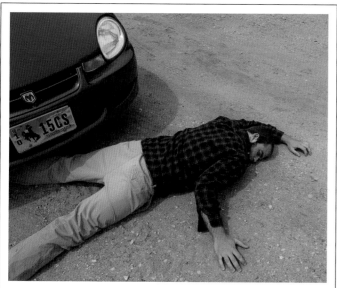

- Vasogenic (vessel-related) shock results when a loss of blood vessel tone causes an increase in the size of the vessels, which produces a loss of blood pressure and inadequate perfusion.

- It can be caused by traumatic injury to the spinal cord and the resulting

failure of nerve messages from the brain to reach the walls of blood vessels.

- It can be caused by a severe allergic reaction.

- It can be caused by sepsis, an overwhelming infection that spreads throughout the body.

YELLOW LIGHT

Emotional stress and pain can cause the signs and symptoms of shock, and, although this patient should be treated, it is extraordinarily rare for this patient's life to be threatened.

Symptoms of Shock

- Rapid and weak heartbeat

- Anxiety, restlessness, disorientation

- Rapid and shallow breathing

- Pale, cool, sweaty skin

- Perhaps nausea, vomiting, dizziness, and/or thirst

TREAT SHOCK 1

Treating mild shock early may prevent it from getting worse

Shock can kill, and, therefore, patients with the signs and symptoms of shock should be treated properly and soon. The sooner you treat for shock, the better your chances of halting or even reversing the problem.

Treatment for shock is aimed at supporting the patient's cardiovascular system: the heart, blood, and vessels that work together to maintain perfusion (see "Shock").

If the patient has a cause of shock that is treatable—such as stopping blood loss or hydrating the dehydrated—your treatment may prevent shock from getting worse. Treat the cause of shock whenever possible.

Keep the patient at rest in a comfortable position. Any form of exercise or physical discomfort increases the workload on the cardiovascular system. In the early stage of shock, patients may prefer to sit comfortably.

Keep the patient warm, such as wrapped in a blanket, and

Treat the Cause

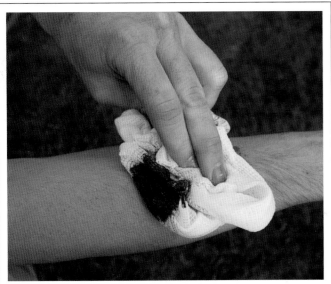

- If you can identify a problem causing the shock, and the problem can be treated, treat it as soon as possible.

- If, for instance, there is serious blood loss, stop it with direct pressure.

- If there is dehydration, provide the patient with plenty of cold, clear fluids. Give the fluids in small amounts to prevent nausea and vomiting.

- If there is a severe allergic reaction, find the patient's injectable epinephrine.

Calm and Reassure

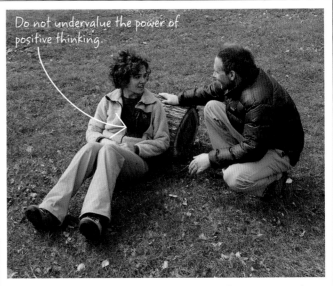

Do not undervalue the power of positive thinking.

- Because the cardiovascular system is challenged by shock, and because emotional stress further challenges the cardiovascular system, all you can do to calm and reassure the patient will be beneficial.

- Use a calm tone of voice, and choose words that are nonthreatening and reassuring.

- Place patients in a position of comfort for them, insulated from the ground if you're outside.

- Patients in the early stages of shock may prefer to sit rather than lie down.

protected from the environment. The challenge to stay warm requires work by the cardiovascular system.

And keep the patient emotionally calm and reassured. Do not underestimate the value of creating and maintaining a positive atmosphere—or, conversely, the potentially devastating effect of a tense, stressful atmosphere.

Protect from Heat Loss

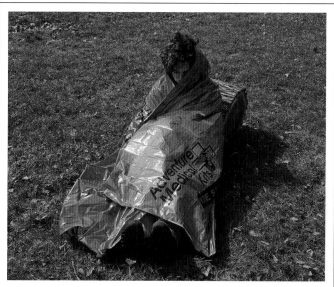

- When a person gets cold, the cardiovascular system increases in involuntary activity as it works to help keep the body warm, carrying blood from warmer body parts to colder body parts.

- Protecting the patient from loss of body heat reduces

the stress that shock is causing the patient.

- Wrap the patient in an insulating covering such as a regular blanket or, outdoors, an emergency/survival blanket.

- Do not leave the patient unattended.

Hydrate

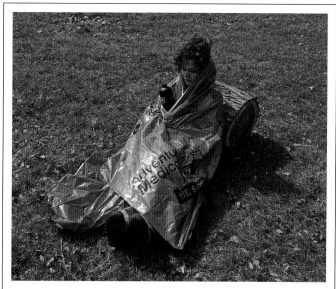

- Even if the cause of shock is not dehydration, almost all patients benefit from hydration.

- If, however, transport to a hospital will be rapid, let the doctor take care of hydration decisions and actions.

- If transportation to a hospital will not be rapid, you can offer the patient cool water to drink.

- The patient needs to be alert enough to swallow, and water should be withheld if it makes the patient nauseous.

BLEEDING & SHOCK

TREAT SHOCK 2

Proper treatment of more serious shock can mean life instead of death

As the patient's cardiovascular system works harder and harder to compensate for the injury or illness causing shock, the heart beats ever faster and weaker, and breathing grows faster and shallower. This patient's treatment needs to be more definitive.

Outdoors, keep the patient lying flat on insulating material to prevent loss of body heat into the ground. Provide enough insulation around the patient to prevent loss of heat into the air. There is less stress on the cardiovascular system when someone is lying down and warm.

You may be able to reduce the workload on the cardiovascular system even more by placing something large and

Lay Patient Down

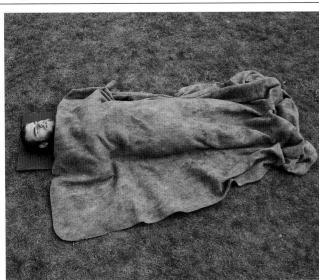

- If the patient shows increasing signs and symptoms of shock—increasingly rapid and weak heartbeat, increasingly shallow breathing, more anxiety, paler skin— keep the patient lying down.

- If you are outdoors, be sure to have the patient lie on insulating material to pre-

vent loss of body heat into the ground.

- Keep the patient covered to prevent loss of body heat into the air.

- The cardiovascular system can keep vital organs perfused more easily when the patient is lying down.

Raise the Legs

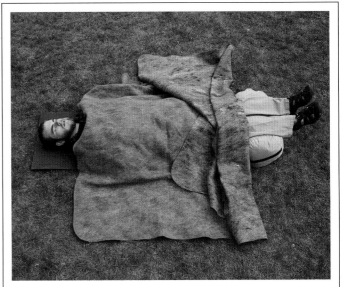

- Blood and the oxygen it carries can be encouraged to circulate with a little more efficiency if the patient's legs are raised.

- Blood that is pumped to the lower extremities returns to the core of the body with less effort.

- Raising the legs too high may be counterproductive, requiring an increased workload on the heart.

- Raise the legs no more than 12 inches, place them on something padded and comfortable.

bulky under the patient's legs to comfortably elevate them 10–12 inches. Simply propping the patient's feet up on something is not recommended due to the decreasing lack of comfort in the legs and back. Comfortably raising the legs a little—not too much—may make the return of blood from the lower extremities less of a chore for the heart.

Because the patient is suffering from an insufficiency of circulating oxygen, supplemental oxygen will usually be of great benefit.

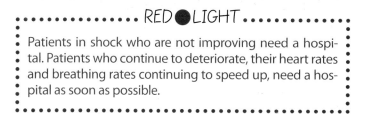

·············· RED ● LIGHT ··············

Patients in shock who are not improving need a hospital. Patients who continue to deteriorate, their heart rates and breathing rates continuing to speed up, need a hospital as soon as possible.

Supplemental Oxygen

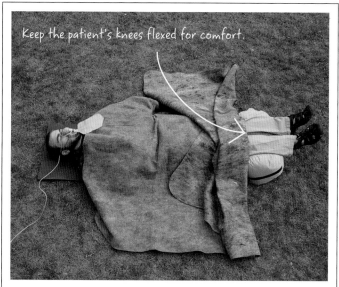

Keep the patient's knees flexed for comfort.

- Because inadequate perfusion means that less than adequate oxygen is getting to the cells of the patient's body, supplemental oxygen could be of great benefit.

- Supplemental oxygen is delivered from a tank that contains 100 percent oxygen, whereas air contains approximately 21 percent oxygen.

- Oxygen is delivered to the patient via a mask.

- Once the oxygen is flowing and the mask is in place, encourage the patient to breathe normally.

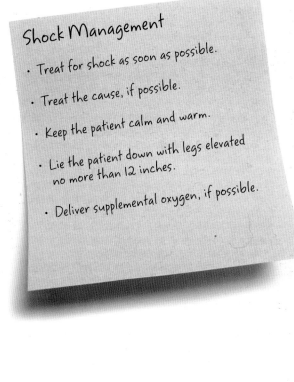

Shock Management

- Treat for shock as soon as possible.

- Treat the cause, if possible.

- Keep the patient calm and warm.

- Lie the patient down with legs elevated no more than 12 inches.

- Deliver supplemental oxygen, if possible.

CHECK THE SPINE 1
A single rescuer can safely roll a patient to check the spine

Injuries to the bones of the spine are potentially devastating for the patient. If the spinal cord is involved, partial or complete paralysis can result. If the cord was not initially involved, improper movement of the patient could cause cord damage.

The first-aid provider is alerted when the mechanism of injury (what happened to the patient) included forces, and the direction in which those forces were applied, that could

have damaged the spine. Mechanisms that could damage the spine include sudden and violent stops, especially vehicle accidents and falls from a height, and especially if the patient's head was involved; excessive rotation, extension, or flexion of the spine, as might happen if a high-speed skier falls without the skis releasing from the bindings; crushing injuries when something heavy falls on the spine; and penetrating spinal injuries such as gunshots or stabbings. As soon

Step 1: Ready to Roll

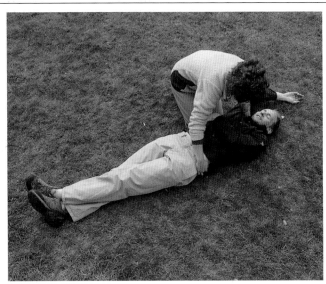

- While keeping one hand on the patient's head to prevent movement of the head and neck, cross the patient's far leg over the near leg, and cross the patient's far arm over the patient's chest.

- Place the patient's near arm alongside the patient's head.

- Slide your hand gently underneath the patient's head.

- Get a firm grip on the patient's far hip. Grasping a bunch of clothing will work, but do not trust a belt loop.

Step 2: Roll

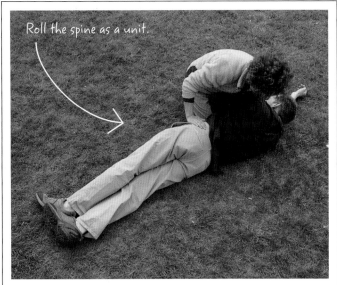

Roll the spine as a unit.

- Count to yourself or out loud with a conscious patient, and roll the patient onto his or her side in one fluid motion. You can ask a conscious patient to tighten the abdominal muscles during the roll.

- You must maintain control

of the patient's head and neck during the roll.

- Keep the spine in line, the neck in line with the back, during the roll.

- Roll the patient slightly forward so the body weight is resting on your thighs.

as you learn the mechanism, and if it could have involved the spine, take control of the patient's head, or have someone else take control, and keep the patient as still as possible. It is usually best to keep the patient still in the position you find that person, unless you are unsure of the patient's breathing and pulse. For instance, you might have to roll a patient from side to back to initiate CPR. But all patients will have to eventually be rolled, either to check the spine or to place them on a pad to insulate them from the ground.

When you perform the roll, cradle the head, take hold of the hip, and make the roll one smooth motion, keeping the patient's spine in line, the head and neck in line with the back. Ask the patient to *not* help.

Step 3: Spine Check

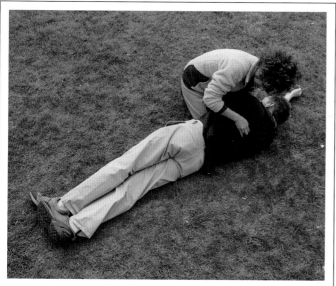

- With one hand still cradling the head, press on every bone of the spine from just below the skull to the lower end of the spine.

- You should press firmly but not aggressively.

- You can press through thin clothing, but you should run your fingers along the spine underneath thick clothing.

- After checking the spine, you should also press on the backs of the shoulders and on the flanks of the patient to check for other injuries.

Step 4: Return to Back

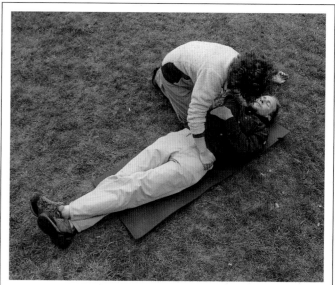

- After you check the spine, patients outdoors will benefit if you roll them back onto a pad or some other insulating material.

- The roll back is the opposite motion of the roll onto a side.

- Keep the patient's head firmly cradled in one hand, and grasp the patient's upper hip with your other hand.

- Roll the patient from side to back with the least amount of motion of the spine itself.

CHECK THE SPINE 2
Two or more rescuers make a spine check easier and safer

When the back of the patient is accessible, the first-aider needs to press firmly but gently down the entire length of the spine. Pain and/or tenderness when touched are the primary indicators of spine damage. You need to check from the base of the skull all the way down to the pelvis.

If the patient must be rolled to assess the spine, several rescuers make the job safer and easier. One rescuer controls the head, and one or two rescuers must kneel beside the patient.

Controlling the patient with rescuers' hands on the head, shoulder, and hip prevents unnecessary movement of the spine during the roll. The rescuer at the patient's head will coordinate the roll. On his or her count ("one, two, three"), the team will roll the patient toward the kneeling rescuers, keeping the spine in line, until the patient rests against the thighs of the rescuers. While the rescuer at the head maintains control, another rescuer presses on each bone of the

Step 1: Ready to Roll

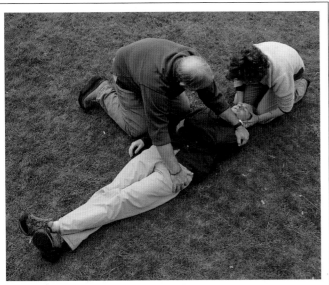

- When two or three first-aid providers are available to roll a patient, it is easier on the patient and the rescuers.

- The rescuer holding the patient's head should be in control of the roll to maximize safety for the patient.

- The head-holder needs to give clear commands, such as "I will count to three, and we will roll when I say 'three.'"

- The head-holder needs to make sure the other rescuers are ready before calling for the roll.

Step 2: Roll and Check

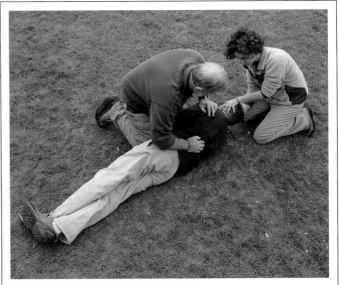

- When the head-holder is assured that the other rescuers are ready, he or she calls for the roll.

- The patient's spine must be kept in line during the roll, the head-holder turning the head to match the roll of the body.

- The head-holder's focus should be on holding the head while another rescuer checks the spine for pain or tenderness.

- If there are two additional rescuers, one should focus on stabilizing the patient while the other checks the spine.

spine, assessing pain and/or tenderness.

Outdoors, all patients need to be placed onto insulating material, such as a sleeping pad, to prevent body heat loss and to provide comfort. The best time to place a pad beneath a patient is when you have rolled the patient to check the spine.

ZOOM

When assessing possible spine damage, ask patients to squeeze your hands with their hands and to move their feet against the resistance of your hands. If they can't, the cord may be involved.

Step 3: Return to Back

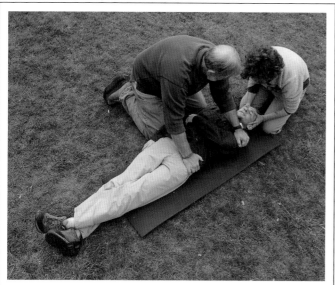

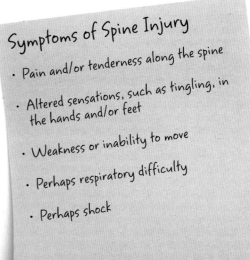

Symptoms of Spine Injury

- Pain and/or tenderness along the spine

- Altered sensations, such as tingling, in the hands and/or feet

- Weakness or inability to move

- Perhaps respiratory difficulty

- Perhaps shock

- In the outdoors, with a patient now on his or her side, it is time to slip a pad or some other insulating material beneath the patient.

- The roll back should once again be under the command of the person holding the patient's head.

- Someone should also check the patient's hands and feet for circulation, sensation, and motion.

- Can the patient move hands and feet, feel when someone touches the hands and feet? Do the hands and feet feel numb or tingly?

SPINE & HEAD

TREAT THE SPINE 1

Proper treatment of a spine-injured patient may prevent permanent damage

If you find yourself in doubt—is the spine damaged? is it not damaged?—it is best for the patient that you assume damage. Proper treatment is critical to prevent further damage.

When you take control of the head, preventing movement of the neck and keeping the patient still, you have actually begun treatment. Manual immobilization is part of it.

As soon as you can, place a cervical collar on the patient to increase resistance to spinal motion. Commercial cervical collars create the best resistance to motion. You can improvise a collar in several ways, which include folding a commercial splint such as the SAM Splint or rolling up a garment such as a fleece jacket (see the following examples).

Manual Stabilization

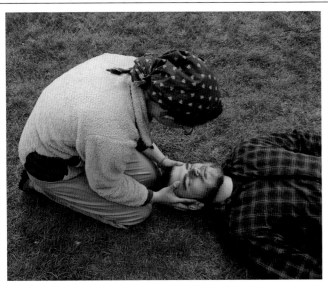

- You have begun treatment of a possible spine injury when you keep a patient from moving.

- If the patient's head lies tilted to one side, it is safe to move it slowly and gently into line with the rest of the spine.

- Movement of the head, however, should *not* cause pain and should *not* meet resistance.

- With the head and neck in line with the rest of the spine, placement of a cervical collar is easier and more effective.

Commercial Collar

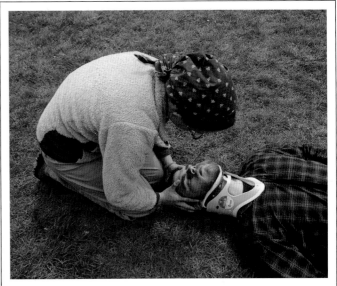

- A cervical collar does not prevent motion of the head and neck, but it does limit the range of motion.

- A commercial cervical collar is slipped beneath the patient's neck and wrapped around in order to cup the chin and prevent the chin

from moving toward the chest.

- A properly sized collar is important. It should not force the chin up and back.

- A properly sized collar does not allow the chin to slip down inside the collar.

To be effective, collars need to go around the patient's neck without impeding breathing, and they cup the patient's chin to prevent chin-to-chest motion. They need to be placed with as little movement of the patient's head as possible.

Placement of a collar does *not* remove the need to keep a stabilizing hand on the head. The final step in prehospital treatment is immobilization of the entire patient on a rigid backboard.

Splint as Collar

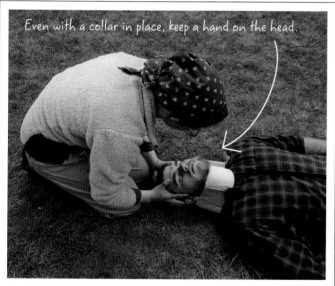

Even with a collar in place, keep a hand on the head.

- Some commercial splints can be folded to create a cervical collar. Although not as effective as a commercial collar, they certainly can be made to work.

- The splint should be folded at both sides of the patient's neck to increase rigidity.

- You will need to fold the splint out at the patient's chin to form a cup for the chin.

- Place something soft in the chin cup to increase the comfort.

Clothing as Collar

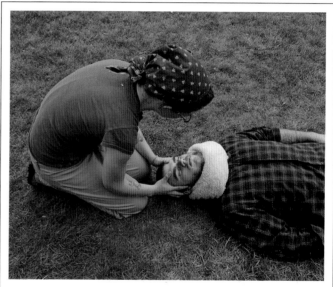

- A long-sleeved garment, such as a fleece jacket, can be used to improvise a cervical collar.

- The garment should be rolled into a tight roll. If the garment is thin, two garments can be rolled together.

- One sleeve should be slipped carefully under the patient's neck, and then the second sleeve, leaving the bulkiest section of the rolled garment under the patient's chin.

- The sleeves should be pulled tight but only enough to keep the collar in place.

SPINE & HEAD

TREAT THE SPINE 2

Movement of a spine-injured patient should be limited as much as possible

Despite the fact that you would rather keep the patient still, there may be times when it is necessary to move the patient over a short distance—to increase safety or comfort. It is critical to do this appropriately.

The safest method of moving a possible spine injury without a backboard requires a team of rescuers. The method is

sometimes referred to as "body elevation and movement" (BEAM). To work best, a BEAM requires someone in charge.

In an emergency situation, a patient can be BEAMed without a cervical collar, but placement of a collar first is preferred.

To perform a BEAM, one rescuer holds the patient's head, and this person is the one in charge. Kneeling on both sides

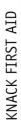

Step 1: Rescuers in Position

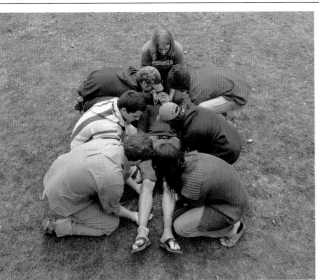

- One rescuer needs to maintain control of the patient's head and neck at all times. This person will be in charge of the lifting and moving.

- The remaining rescuers need to kneel on both sides of the patient, gently working their hands underneath the patient's body.

- The strongest rescuers are best positioned at the patient's upper torso, providing adequate support for the patient's spine.

- With five rescuers, one is usually enough to lift the patient's legs.

Step 2: Lifting and Moving

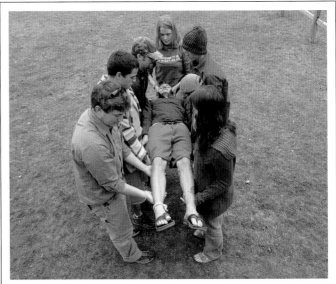

- The rescuer at the patient's head needs to be sure that everyone is prepared to lift and that everyone understands the carrying plan.

- The kneeling rescuers should be prepared to lift with their legs and not with their backs to prevent injury to themselves.

- Lifting the patient, on the head-holder's command, needs to be as smooth as possible.

- At the head-holder's command, the patient should be moved with short, shuffling steps to avoid stumbling.

of the patient are four to six other rescuers, and these people gently work their hands underneath the patient. On the command of the head-holder, the rescuers stand as a team, maintaining the patient's spine in line.

Movement with the patient must be slow and coordinated. It is strongly recommended that the rescuers step in unison and shuffle their feet, avoiding crossing their feet as they step (to reduce the chance of stumbling).

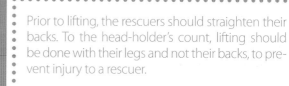

ZOOM

Prior to lifting, the rescuers should straighten their backs. To the head-holder's count, lifting should be done with their legs and not their backs, to prevent injury to a rescuer.

Step 3: Lowering the Patient

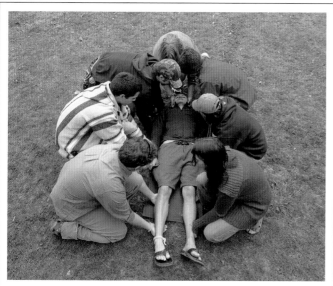

- Carry the patient feet first to prevent the head-holder from having to back up.

- When the new location is reached, it is best to have some sort of insulating material ready to lower the patient onto.

- If the patient will be lowered onto a backboard, have someone slip the backboard into position under the patient to prevent the rescuer from having to step over it.

- At the command of the head-holder, the patient is lowered, once again in one fluid motion.

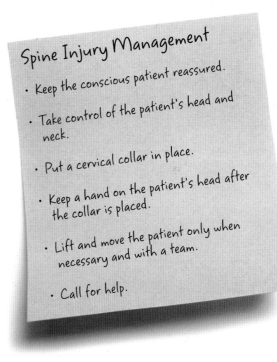

Spine Injury Management

- Keep the conscious patient reassured.

- Take control of the patient's head and neck.

- Put a cervical collar in place.

- Keep a hand on the patient's head after the collar is placed.

- Lift and move the patient only when necessary and with a team.

- Call for help.

SPINE & HEAD

CHECK THE HEAD

Injuries that cause the brain to swell can end a life in a brief time

Scalp lacerations (cuts) and blows that produce "goose-egg" bumps are relatively minor—unless the blow is forceful enough to damage the brain. There is simply almost no room inside a head for the brain to swell, so swelling may cause death.

Check the head for obvious damage: deep cuts, bumps, and bruises. Finding damage will be your first clue. Press gently over the entire surface of the head, checking for depressions in the skull. A skull fracture is a second and serious sign. Skull fractures, however, may exist without obvious depressions. Bruising around the eyes ("raccoon eyes") and behind the ears ("Battle's sign") are indications of a skull fracture. You may also see clear fluid or blood leaking from the ears or the nose.

But the brain can swell without a skull fracture. An obvious sign is a change in the mental status of patients. They tend

Checking the Head

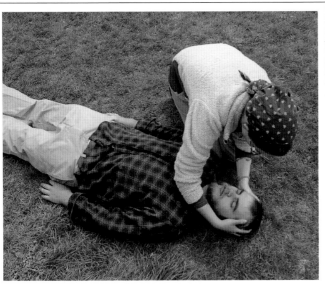

- Any severe blow to a patient's head could cause a brain injury, especially if the blow caused a period of unconsciousness.

- Inspect the head carefully with your hands spread wide, pressing gently but firmly. You will need to lift the head slightly to check the back of the head.

- Check for bumps, bruises, and open wounds.

- Be especially wary of a depression in the skull, evidence that the skull has been fractured.

Raccoon Eyes

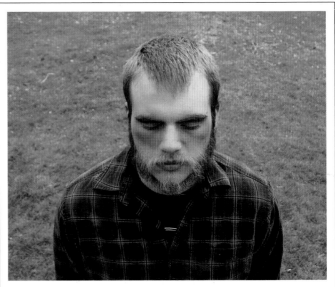

- Bruising and sometimes swelling around both eyes after a blow to the head are called "raccoon eyes."

- The patient may appear to have two black eyes, but raccoon eyes always develop in both eyes and not just one eye.

- Raccoon eyes are most often caused by a skull fracture followed by blood filling the soft tissue around the eyes.

- Sometimes hours pass after the blow to the head before raccoon eyes develop.

to grow disoriented, irritable, and combative, and they may exhibit bizarre behavior. They may grow drowsy. Patients may complain of severe headache or pressure inside the head; nausea, with or without vomiting; vision difficulties; and tingling or loss of feeling in part of their body. Their pupils may become unequal in size.

Any patient who lapses into unconsciousness is in serious condition indeed.

••••••••••••••• RED ● LIGHT ••••••••••••••

If you see signs and symptoms indicating that the brain could be swelling and/or that the skull is fractured, you need an ambulance and a hospital as soon as possible.

Battle's Sign

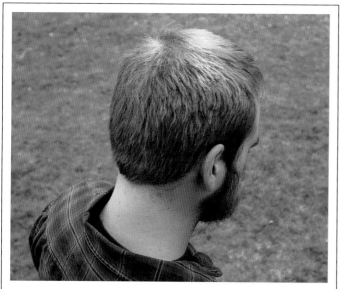

- Battle's sign—bruising behind and slightly below the ear—is another indication of a fracture of the skull.

- When checking behind the ears, do not lift and turn the patient's head.

- Sometimes hours, even days, pass before Battle's sign develops, but a bloody discharge may leak from the ears shortly after the injury.

- All patients with indications of a head injury require transport to a hospital as soon as possible.

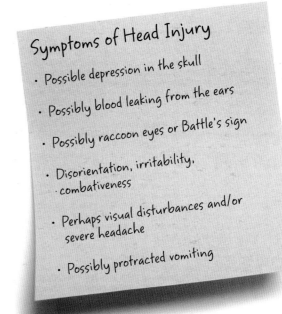

Symptoms of Head Injury

- Possible depression in the skull

- Possibly blood leaking from the ears

- Possibly raccoon eyes or Battle's sign

- Disorientation, irritability, combativeness

- Perhaps visual disturbances and/or severe headache

- Possibly protracted vomiting

SPINE & HEAD

45

TREAT THE HEAD

Proper treatment of a head injury may provide enough care to prevent permanent damage

For seriously brain-injured patients, unfortunately, there is little to be done in the field. Salvation lies in early recognition and rapid access to definitive care. You may, however, be able to "buy some time."

Any drowsy patient is best placed in a stable side position, a position that makes it easier to breathe. Patients on their back may be gently rolled into the side position, with care given to keep the spine in line (see "Treat the Spine 1"). Once a patient is rolled, a pillow under the head will help keep the spine in line. You are concerned about the spine because forceful blows to the head occasionally damage the neck.

Any patient being treated for brain injury is best left in a

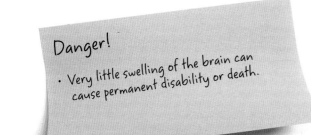

Danger!
• Very little swelling of the brain can cause permanent disability or death.

Stable Side Position

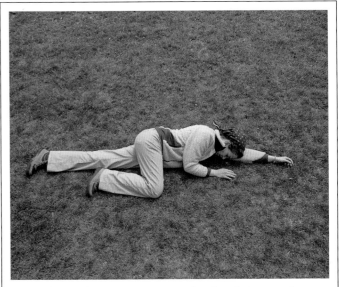

- Lethargy and excessive drowsiness are common with an injury to the brain, and seizures are possible. Sleep may be undeniable.

- For these reasons, patients positioned on their backs may have difficulty maintaining their airways and may inhale vomit.

- Gently roll these patients into a stable side position (the recovery position) as pictured.

- Placing a small pillow under the head provides comfort and helps keep the patient's airway in line and open.

stable side position if he or she must be left alone for any time.

Brain injuries cause the brain to suffer from oxygen deprivation—so supplemental oxygen, when available, will be of great benefit.

Despite complaints of a headache, the patient is best denied pain medication. Painkillers can mask signs and symptoms, and some over-the-counter medications, such as aspirin and ibuprofen, could increase the rate of bleeding in the head and thus the swelling.

•••••••••••••••• RED ● LIGHT ••••••••••••
Any blow to the head that causes unconsciousness, even for a short period, needs to be evaluated by a physician. The speed of the need is relative to the signs and symptoms.

Supplemental Oxygen

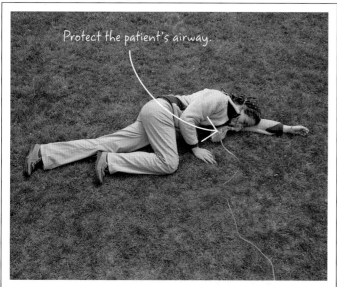

Protect the patient's airway.

- A brain injury often causes the brain to get less oxygen than it needs, so supplemental oxygen may be of great benefit.

- If supplemental oxygen is available, it should be delivered at the highest flow rate possible.

- Patients forcefully knocked unconscious could also have sustained a neck injury and should be managed accordingly.

- First aid, however, does little good, and rapid access to professional transport of the patient is critical.

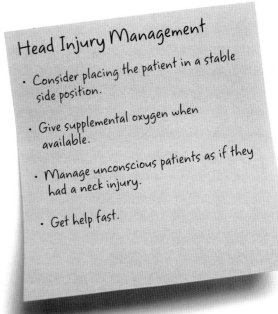

Head Injury Management

- Consider placing the patient in a stable side position.

- Give supplemental oxygen when available.

- Manage unconscious patients as if they had a neck injury.

- Get help fast.

SPINE & HEAD

CHECK THE CHEST

The sooner you discover a chest injury, the better your chance of helping

An injury to the chest could lead to breathing difficulty and then to a critical patient. The sooner you recognize a serious chest injury and treat it, the better the chances for the patient.

With all patients, develop the habit of asking if they are having any difficulty breathing. Ask as soon as possible after arriving at their side.

With all patients who have been involved in an accident, develop the habit of pressing in on both sides of the chest simultaneously and asking them to take a deep breath. It's also a good idea to press on the sternum with the side of your hand. Patients with unrecognized chest injuries will complain of pain, either upon inhaling and/or in response to your pressure.

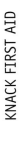

Checking the Chest 1

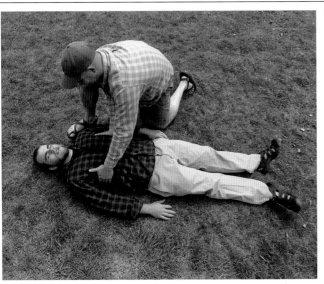

- Checking the chest often begins with you asking patients if they are having any difficulty breathing.

- Then ask patients to take a deep breath to see if the effort changes anything.

- If you are pressing in on both sides of the patient's chest at the same time, the patient must inhale against minor resistance, increasing the chance of noticing any pain.

- You may check twice, the first time with your hands high near the armpits, the second time with your hands lower on the rib cage.

Checking the Chest 2

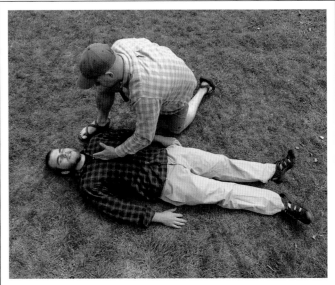

- Additionally, you can press on the patient's sternum (breastbone) to check for an injury.

- Use the side of your hand, similar to a karate chop, to avoid being overly intrusive.

- A chest injury may also be indicated by a patient who "splints" the injury by pressing a hand or arm supportively against the injury site.

- The greater the amount of pain the patient reports, the greater your concern will be.

If a patient claims chest pain, or if you see blood on the shirt or blouse, you need to check beneath the garment, taking a look at bare skin.

Chest injuries could be indicated by any combination of pain, wounds, redness or bruising, or a section of chest that does not move in concert with the rest of the chest on inhalation. Patients may complain of difficulty breathing without any visible evidence of injury. And patients may "guard" or protect a part of their chest—another response to injury.

 ZOOM

When pressing on the chest with the flat of your hands to check for injury, keep your hands spread wide to cover as much area as possible.

Take a Look

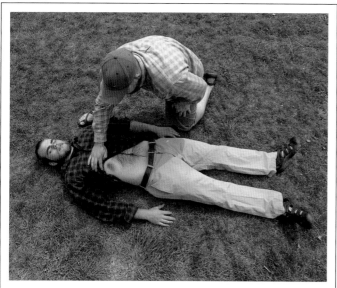

- If a patient reports pain in the chest or if the patient reports difficulty breathing after an injury to the chest, you must take a look immediately.

- You must remove enough clothing to look at skin level.

- You must also take a look at skin level if you see blood and/or tears in clothing that were caused by the injury, even if the patient reports no pain.

- Remember: First aid for almost all injuries is administered at skin level.

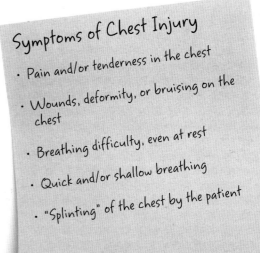

Symptoms of Chest Injury

- Pain and/or tenderness in the chest
- Wounds, deformity, or bruising on the chest
- Breathing difficulty, even at rest
- Quick and/or shallow breathing
- "Splinting" of the chest by the patient

49

RIB INJURY

Injuries to the bones of the chest range from mild to deadly

Broken ribs and collarbones (clavicles) account for the vast majority of chest injuries, and, although sometimes disturbingly painful, they are seldom serious. Some chest fractures, however, can be devastatingly serious.

Adults normally breathe about twelve to twenty times per minute effortlessly and painlessly. Fractured ribs, because of the pain, cause the patient to breathe with shallow breaths. By breathing with shallow breaths, the patient should be able to moderate the pain. Some patients require no special treatment. Others will feel better with the arm on the affected side secured in a sling-and-swathe (see "Splint an Upper Arm").

But if two or more consecutive ribs are broken in two or more places, the result could be a *flail*, a section of chest wall no longer attached via bones to the rest of the chest. Flails are often indicated by the "free-floating" section of chest moving in opposition to the rest of the chest during breathing. A

Fractures

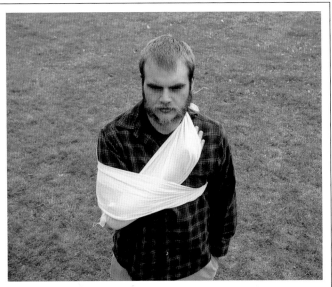

- Broken ribs and broken collarbones are the most common chest injuries, and they are usually not serious.

- You may or may not see bruising at the injury site, but you will elicit pain when you press gently on the site of the fracture.

- Prior to transportation, secure the arm on the injured side with a sling-and-swathe (pictured).

- The sling needs to cup the elbow and hold it securely up so the patient can let the arm rest in the sling.

Improvisation

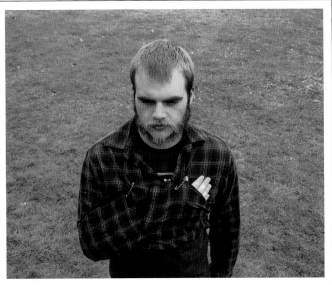

- Ambulances often carry commercial slings, and first-aid kits may contain large, triangular bandages used to create a sling-and-swathe.

- With two safety pins, you can fold a patient's shirt up over an arm and pin it in place to create an improvised sling (pictured).

- This works with almost any shirt, including a T-shirt.

- To swathe an improvised sling, you can put a jacket on the patient and zip it up.

large flail makes it extremely difficult to breath. You can tape a bulky pad over the flail and have the patient lie with the injured side down, and this might help breathing.

Flail

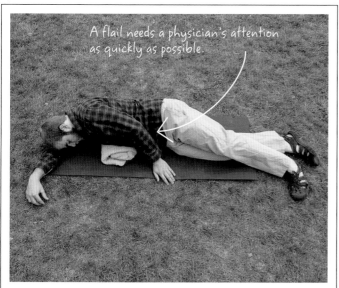

A flail needs a physician's attention as quickly as possible.

- A flail is two or more consecutive ribs broken in two or more places.

- The flail, a "free-floating" section of the chest wall, does not move or appears to move in opposition to the rest of the chest when the patient inhales.

- This is a serious injury requiring rapid access to a hospital.

- While waiting for the ambulance, patients may breathe better if you lay them on their injured side with a thick pad pressing on the flail.

Chest Fracture Management

- Sling-and-swathe the arm on the injured side for rib and collarbone fractures.

- Consider placing patients with flails onto their sides with a pad under the flail.

- If transport is delayed, consider painkilling drugs.

- Give supplemental oxygen, if available.

51

LUNG INJURY

All injuries to the lungs must be managed quickly and appropriately

Injuries to the chest that damage a lung often cause great difficulty breathing and sometimes a possibility of death.

A fractured rib may involve a bone fragment stabbing inward to puncture a lung. Air escaping the lung on inhalation can collect in the chest outside the lung, creating a *closed pneumothorax*. Over time the "dead air" in the chest cavity can grow in size. The patient will experience increasing difficulty breathing, especially difficulty taking a deep breath, as the trapped air takes up more and more breathing room.

More often than not, a pneumothorax reaches a point where it gets no worse. But it can worsen until the patient is unable to breathe adequately, a condition known as a "tension pneumothorax," a life-threatening chest injury.

If the chest has been opened by a penetrating object, the resulting hole may make noise when the patient breathes. This is an *open pneumothorax*, and the air being sucked in

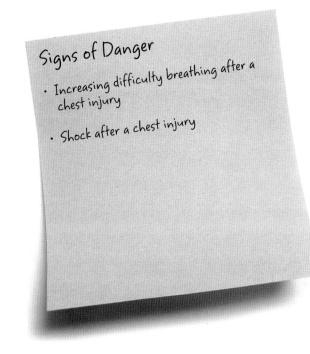

Signs of Danger

• Increasing difficulty breathing after a chest injury

• Shock after a chest injury

Closed Chest Injury

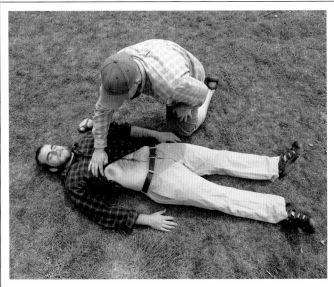

• A severe blow to the chest wall can cause damage to the underlying lung tissue.

• You will almost always see an indication, such as bruising of the chest wall, at the injury site.

• The most important indication of lung injury is increasing difficulty breathing.

• Create a sling-and-swathe for the arm on the injured side, and place the patient in the position that provides the most comfort while waiting for transport.

through the wound does nothing to sustain life.

You must plug the hole immediately. Your hand, preferably gloved, will work, and quick action could prove life-saving. Then cover the wound with an occlusive dressing—something that lets no air or water pass through. Clean plastic will work. Tape this dressing in place on all four sides. An open pneumothorax can become a tension pneumothorax.

Open Chest Injury

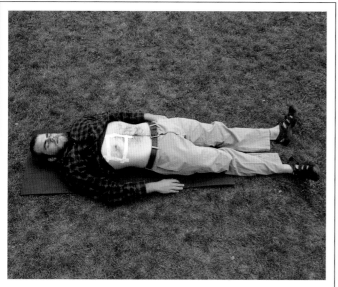

- When an object penetrates the chest wall and damages underlying lung tissue, the patient has an open chest injury.

- The wound often bubbles or "sucks" when the patient breathes.

- Immediately cover this wound with your hand until you can replace your hand with an occlusive dressing, a dressing that allows no air to pass through.

- The dressing can be a piece of clean plastic. Tape it down securely on all four sides.

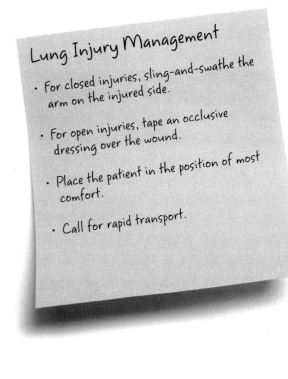

Lung Injury Management

- For closed injuries, sling-and-swathe the arm on the injured side.

- For open injuries, tape an occlusive dressing over the wound.

- Place the patient in the position of most comfort.

- Call for rapid transport.

CHECK THE ABDOMEN
Many organs and major vessels make assessment complicated

It is practically impossible to tell from the outside what sort of damage has occurred inside a patient's abdominal cavity. You can, however, learn to detect a serious injury.

Observe the patient's body position. Although pain is not always a reliable indicator of the seriousness of an injury, a patient who lies still with legs drawn up into a fetal position is often assuming a posture that minimizes serious pain.

Look at the abdomen with the patient lying down. A normal abdomen is gently rounded and symmetrical. Look for distention and/or an irregularly shaped abdomen, both of which may indicate a serious injury. Look for bruises, penetrating wounds, or obvious injuries, and don't forget to check the flanks, where damage to the kidneys might be indicated. Find out as much as you can about any object that has penetrated the abdomen.

Press gently in all four quadrants of the abdomen. Watch for

Checking the Abdomen

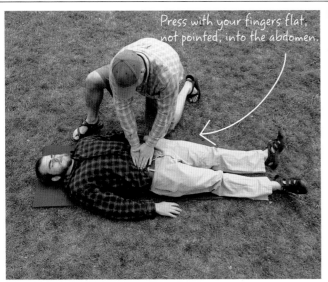

Press with your fingers flat, not pointed, into the abdomen.

- The abdominal region contains a large number of organs and large blood vessels that can be injured by blunt or penetrating trauma.

- These organs and vessels lie completely or partially within one of four abdominal quadrants.

- The four quadrants are created by imagining two lines drawn through the belly button, one line horizontal, the other line vertical.

- Press gently with flat fingers on all four quadrants to check the whole abdomen.

Check the Pelvis

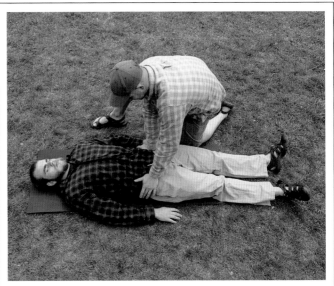

- Fractures of the pelvis are often associated with damage to organs and/or large blood vessels in the lower abdominal region.

- It is possible for the patient to bleed to death internally from a fracture of the pelvis.

- Check the pelvis by cupping the two pelvic crests (pictured) and pressing gently down and then in.

- If you can tie a wide band securely around a fractured pelvis, it may slow internal bleeding while you wait for transport.

a pain response. Normal abdomens are soft and not tender to palpation. Feel for rigid muscles, lumps, and pain specific to a local spot, all of which may be signs of injury.

Take a Look

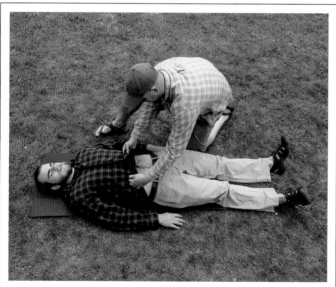

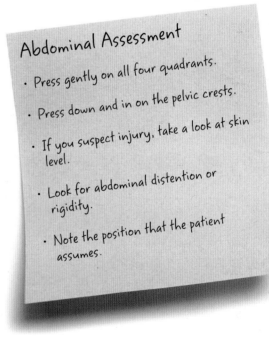

Abdominal Assessment

- Press gently on all four quadrants.

- Press down and in on the pelvic crests.

- If you suspect injury, take a look at skin level.

- Look for abdominal distention or rigidity.

- Note the position that the patient assumes.

- If you suspect damage to the abdominal region, remove enough clothing to inspect the abdomen.

- With a patient lying on the back, a normal abdomen is flat or gently rounded.

- If the abdomen is abnormally distended and/or rigid to your touch, it may indicate internal damage.

- If the patient refuses to straighten the legs or insists that a side position with the legs curled is more comfortable, it may indicate internal damage.

CLOSED ABDOMINAL INJURY
A forceful blow to the abdomen may cause an internal rupture

The abdominal cavity holds both hollow and solid organs.

Ruptured hollow organs may release substances into the abdomen such as stomach acid, digested food, or bacteria. Hollow organs' contents are highly irritating. *Peritonitis*, an inflammatory reaction in the abdominal cavity, will probably develop with pain—described as sharp, stabbing, or burning—increasing and spreading throughout the abdomen. Pulse and respirations quicken. The muscles of the abdomen often become increasingly rigid and distended.

Because solid organs bleed when ruptured, and because blood is less irritating than hollow organ contents, the signs and symptoms of peritonitis may not appear. The signs and symptoms of shock may appear (see "Shock"). You should also see increasing rigidity and distention. Pain may increase. Be aware that pain from a damaged liver may refer to the right shoulder, and pain from a damaged spleen may refer to

Diaphragm

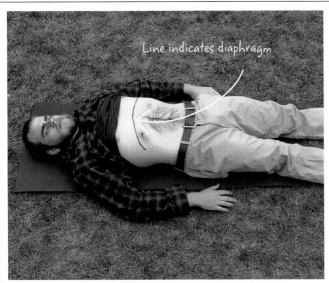

Line indicates diaphragm

- The diaphragm is a dome-shaped muscle that separates the chest cavity from the abdominal cavity.

- The top of the "dome" is near the bottom of the sternum, and the bottom of the "dome" attaches near the bottom of the rib cage.

- But some abdominal organs, such as the liver, spleen, and kidneys, are partially or completely underneath the rib cage.

- Injuries to the lower ribs may involve the upper abdominal organs.

Right Upper Quadrant

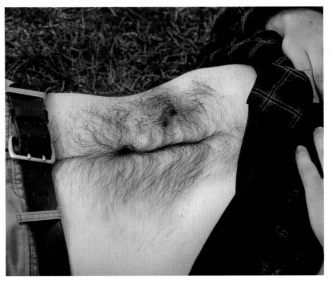

- The right upper quadrant of the abdomen contains most of the liver, the gall-bladder, the right kidney, part of the colon, and part of the pancreas.

- Severe blunt trauma to the front or side of this quadrant can cause significant bleeding from the liver.

- Severe blunt trauma to the side or back of this quadrant can cause significant bleeding from the kidney.

- Internal bleeding can be significant enough to cause shock.

the left shoulder. Threat to life may be immediate.

With any abdominal injury, anticipate nausea and vomiting. Over time, blood may appear in the vomit (often looking like "coffee grounds"), in the urine (often appearing pale pink), or in the stool (often described as "black and tarry"), depending on where the damage occurred. Over time, a fever may develop.

Stay alert to the possibility of vomiting. Generally, treat for shock.

Left Upper Quadrant

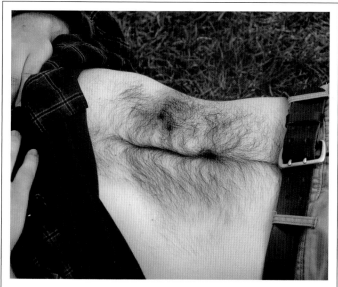

- The left upper quadrant contains some of the liver, the spleen, the left kidney, part of the pancreas, part of the colon, and most of the stomach.

- Severe blunt trauma to the front of this quadrant can cause rupture of the stomach, especially if the stomach is full on impact, or bleeding from the liver.

- Severe blunt trauma to the front or side of this quadrant can cause bleeding from the spleen.

- Internal bleeding can be significant enough to cause shock.

Treatment

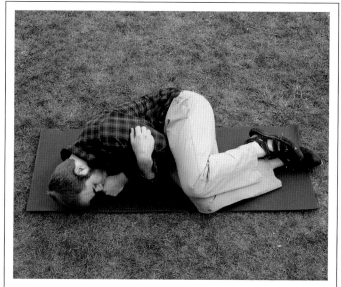

- Allow the patient to assume the position that provides the most comfort.

- This position is typically on a side with the knees flexed and the legs drawn up—what may be called the "fetal position."

- Protect the patient from loss of body heat.

- Give nothing by mouth unless transport of the patient will be significantly delayed, in which case give cool, clear fluids (if the fluids do not cause nausea).

CHEST & ABDOMINAL

OPEN ABDOMINAL INJURY

Wounds that penetrate the abdominal cavity may cause extensive damage

The immediate seriousness of any penetrating abdominal injury, as with blunt trauma, is determined by what got damaged inside and how bad it's bleeding. Over time the risk of infection is very high. General assessment and treatment of the patient are the same as with a patient suffering blunt abdominal trauma. Specific treatment will vary somewhat

depending on the soft tissue involvement. External bleeding should be controlled as much as possible. Wounds should be cleaned and bandaged (see "Wounds & Burns"). Impaled objects, in almost all cases, should be stabilized in place with clean, bulky padding.

An *evisceration* is a specific type of penetrating injury that

Abdominal Wound

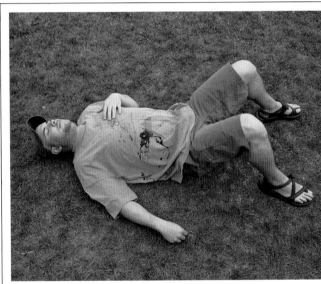

- Wounds to the abdominal region are often indicated by blood on the clothing and often by tears in the clothing.

- Deep wounds often damage the organs and great vessels that lie in that particular quadrant of the abdomen.

- The indication of internal bleeding will be a patient progressively deteriorating into shock—increasing pulse, increasingly rapid and shallow breathing, and increasingly pale and sweaty skin.

- Rapidly transport patient to a medical facility.

Abdominal Wound Treatment

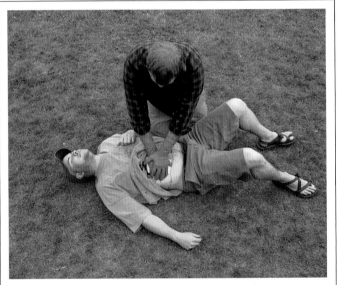

- The wound must be immediately exposed at skin level.

- Press a bulky dressing, a trauma dressing from a first-aid kit, or a thick pad of clean clothing firmly into the wound. Maintain the pressure until help arrives.

- Unfortunately, this may not be enough to adequately slow the flow of internal bleeding.

- If you see the signs and symptoms of shock, treat the patient as best you can for shock.

opens the abdomen and lets intestines protrude. In short-term care, cover the exposed bowels with sterile dressings soaked in disinfected water. Check the dressings every two hours to make sure they stay moist. Cover the moist dressings with thick, dry dressings. In long-term care, over several hours, the exposed intestines will do better if they are flushed clean with clean water and "teased" back inside by gently pulling the wound open. If teasing does not work, you may have to gently push the exposed loops of intestine back inside the abdominal cavity. Then clean and bandage the wound.

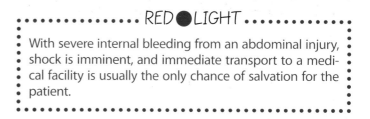
Gunshot Wounds

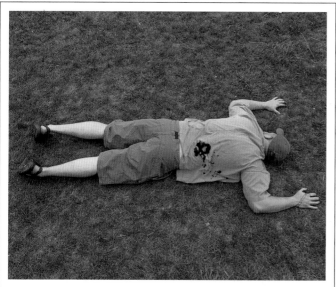

- The bullet from a gun often enters with enough force to pass entirely through the patient, causing extreme damage to internal tissues.

- If you are treating a patient for a gunshot wound, you must inspect both sides of the patient to check for an exit wound.

- Pressure with a bulky dressing must be applied to both entrance and exit wounds.

- Once again, rapid transport of the patient is of the utmost importance.

Abdominal Impalements

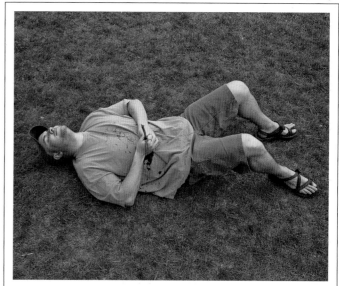

- No attempt should be made to remove an object that is embedded in the abdominal region.

- Any movement of the object may make the injuries to internal organs worse.

- You can apply a bulky dressing around the object and press gently but firmly on the dressing if bleeding is significant.

- Call as soon as possible for help. Place soft, bulky padding around the object to prevent movement, and use tape or strips of soft material to hold the padding in place.

CHEST & ABDOMINAL

CHECK JOINTS & BONES

Injuries to joints, bones, and muscles are among the most common

Bones, muscles, the tendons that attach muscles to bones, and the ligaments that attach bones to bones comprise most of the musculoskeletal system—and injuries to this system are among the most common reasons why someone needs first aid. The first-aid provider often does not know for sure what injury has occurred, but strains are tears in muscles and tendons, sprains are tears in ligaments, bones break (fracture), and dislocations occur when bones are forced out of their normal alignment at a joint.

To properly assess, you need to LAF (look, ask, feel) at the injury.

Look, at skin level, for swelling and discoloration (bruising). How quickly the injury swells and how badly it discolors are indications of the degree of damage.

Ask about the amount of pain the patient is experiencing. Although pain is subjective, it is also a primary indicator of

Sprains

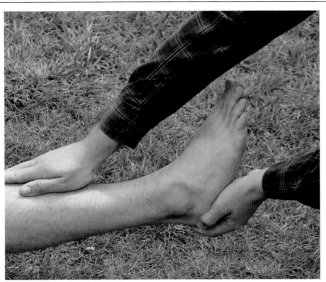

- Sprains are injuries to the ligaments that hold bones to bones.

- A first-degree sprain, the most common, involves overstretching of ligaments but little or no actual tearing of a ligament. There is some pain, a little discoloration, and perhaps a little swelling.

- A second-degree sprain involves partial tearing of ligaments, indicated by pain, swelling, and discoloration.

- A third-degree sprain involves serious ligament tears, often complete tears, and most patients are unable to move the damaged joint.

Fractures

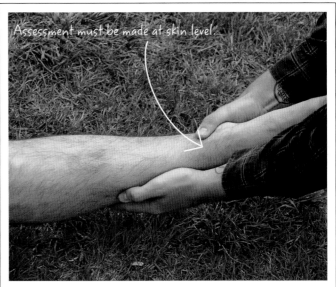

Assessment must be made at skin level.

- Breaks in bones vary in size and shape and include transverse, oblique, spiral, and comminuted fractures.

- The forces involved are usually greater than the forces involved in sprains, and there is typically a great deal of pain.

- You will often see bruising and swelling near the fracture site and perhaps deformity if the bone is unstable.

- Muscles near the fracture spasm, and you can often feel the muscle tightness near the fracture site.

damage. Has the patient suffered similar pain before, and, if so, what was the cause?

Feel, or press firmly but gently, at the site of the injury. If you elicit pain at a specific point (point tenderness), it is another sign of injury.

• • • • • • • • • • • • • RED ● LIGHT • • • • • • • • • • • • •

If you are unsure whether the injury is mild or severe, it is most often in the best interest of the patient to treat it as severe—and get the patient to a hospital.

Dislocations

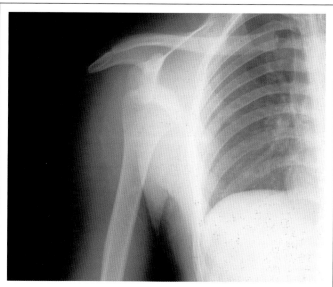

- A dislocation occurs when a joint is forced out of its normal bone-to-bone relationship.

- Patients often know they have a dislocation and typically report a lot of pain, especially with larger joints.

- At skin level, you will usu-ally see obvious deformity, especially when you com-pare the injured joint with the opposite joint on the uninjured side.

- The dislocated joint will have a reduced range of motion, especially com-pared with the opposite uninjured joint.

Symptoms of Musculoskeletal Injury

- Pain

- Point tenderness

- Bruising (discoloration)

- Swelling, deformity, other lack of symmetry

- Guarding (overprotectiveness by the patient)

R.I.C.E.

Rest, ice, compression, and elevation are useful immediately and over time

Most musculoskeletal injuries benefit from R.I.C.E. (rest, ice, compression, and elevation). R.I.C.E. reduces pain and swelling, and, because it reduces swelling, it may actually speed healing. It should be applied as soon as possible after the injury, but R.I.C.E. works even days after the injury.

"Rest" means keeping the patient at rest. If possible, avoid all movements by the injured body part.

"Ice" refers to cooling the injury. But you don't need ice. You can use a chemical cold pack or snow in a plastic bag (when available), or wrap the injury in water-soaked cotton on a warm day and allow evaporation to do the cooling. Apply "ice" for no more than twenty to thirty minutes.

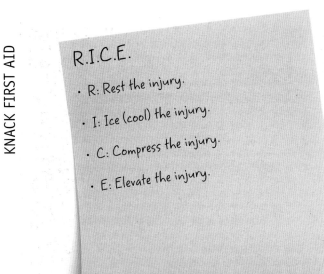

R.I.C.E.

- R: Rest the injury.
- I: Ice (cool) the injury.
- C: Compress the injury.
- E: Elevate the injury.

Compression

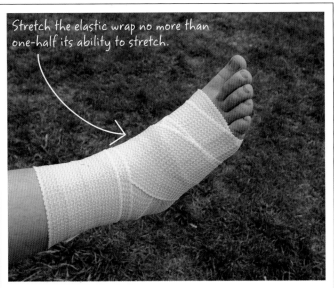

Stretch the elastic wrap no more than one-half its ability to stretch.

- Adequate compression requires an elastic wrap that you can apply evenly around the site of the injury.

- Start applying the elastic wrap away from the heart and move toward the heart.

- Apply the elastic wrap at approximately 50 percent of its ability to stretch. A wrap applied too tightly can cut off necessary circulation.

- Monitor the patient after applying the wrap to make sure that swelling that may continue under the wrap does not make the wrap become too tight.

"Compression" requires an elastic wrap. Apply it toward the heart, for example, from the toes up or from the fingers up. Compression should not be too tight because it can cut off too much circulation.

"Elevation" means keeping the injured body part slightly—and comfortably—above the level of the patient's heart.

There is little danger of overdoing R.I.C.E. as long as you allow sufficient time for normal circulation to return between applications. You could use R.I.C.E. safely at least six or seven times a day.

Ice

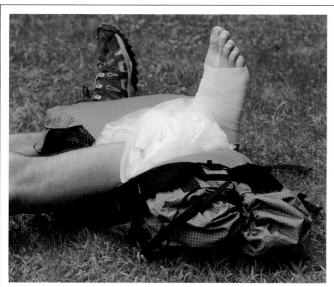

- Although ice works well, it is not your only option for cooling an injury site.

- Gel packs kept in a freezer until needed and disposable chemical ice packs stored at room temperature until needed work as well as ice.

- Ice and other cold packs are too cold to apply directly to skin. Wrap them in a thin, dry cloth first.

- A wet cotton cloth applied to skin cools an injury via evaporation.

Elevation

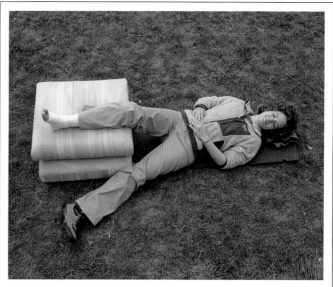

- Elevation works to decrease swelling by encouraging blood that flows to an injury site to flow easily out again.

- The injury site need be elevated to only slightly higher than the patient's heart.

- Elevate the injury in a position that is comfortable for the patient.

- If a lower leg is injured, do not elevate the foot by placing something under the heel, a position that eventually causes stress on the knee.

SPLINT A LOWER ARM
A good splint provides safety and comfort for the patient

A properly applied splint reduces the chance of further injury and provides increased comfort to the patient. A splint should be applied to any injury that could be a fracture. And when you are unsure, apply a splint.

Prior to applying a splint, check for circulation, sensation, and mobility below the injury. If the skin below the injury is colder or paler in color than the skin of the uninjured arm (or leg), you want to know before you splint. If there is numbness

or tingling, you want to know before you splint. Remove rings, watches, and bracelets before splinting.

Prepare the splinting material prior to moving the limb, and move the limb as little as possible during splinting.

The first part of a splint is soft material used to pad the injury site and any natural hollows such as the wrist area of a lower arm. Place a soft pad in the patient's palm so that the hand is not pressed flat. Padding hollows increases comfort and

Step 1: Padding

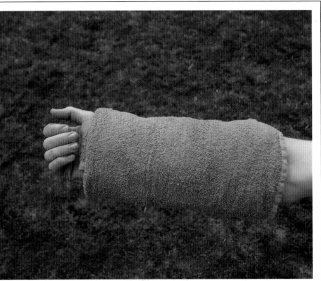

- Padding is the first step in the creation of an adequate splint.

- Padding provides comfort as well as protection to a broken bone.

- It should be soft material that you wrap entirely around the arm, providing comfort where the arm will lie against the rigid support and protection from all directions.

- It will fill the natural voids, such as at the wrist, when the arm is secured to the rigid support.

Step 2: Rigid Support

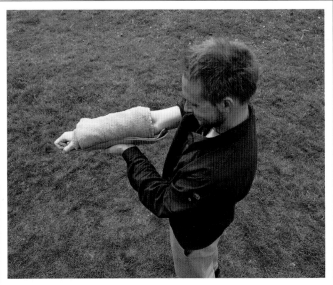

- The part of a splint that provides rigid support needs to be long enough to involve the joints above and below a fracture.

- If the fracture is near a joint, the support needs to be long enough to support the bones above and below the joint.

- Although commercial products are available, you can use many things, including boards, sticks, and rolled newspaper.

- Place the rigid support beneath the arm, not to the side of the arm.

prevents the limb from shifting around inside the splint.

Next, attach the limb to something stiff or rigid. You can use an elastic wrap or strips of any soft material. Splint securely but not so tightly that circulation is cut off. The stiff or rigid material should immobilize the wrist and the elbow of a lower arm.

Finally, the lower arm should be secured in a sling-and-swathe. The sling supports the arm at about the level of the patient's heart. Without sling material, you can fold the patient's shirt up over the arm and safety pin it in place. A swathe is soft material that ties the slung arm to the patient's chest, further preventing unnecessary movement.

After splinting, check circulation and sensation in the hand once again to make sure your splint is not too tight.

Step 3: Attaching the Support

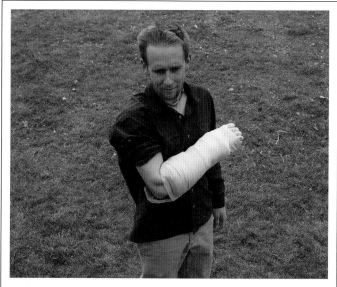

- The rigid support needs to be secured to the arm with strips of soft material or elastic wraps.

- If you are tying knots in strips of material, do not place a knot directly over the site of the injury.

- Elastic wraps work especially well because you can evenly disperse the pressure along the arm.

- Elastic wraps hold the arm to the rigid support with less movement than do strips of material.

Step 4: Sling-and-Swathe

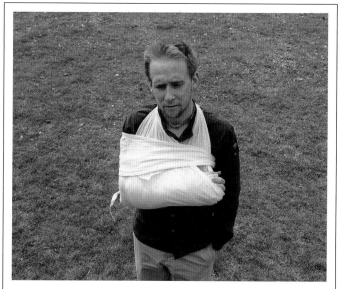

- A sling holds the arm up, and a swathe holds the arm to the chest wall.

- Many first-aid kits include a large triangular bandage that can be used as a sling or a swathe.

- The sling should hold the arm at approximately the level of the patient's heart.

- You can improvise a sling-and-swathe by folding the patient's shirt up over the arm and securing it in place with safety pins.

SPLINT AN UPPER ARM
The basic sling-and-swathe, with variations, works for upper and lower arms

All skilled first-aid providers can properly apply a sling-and-swathe and/or improvise a sling-and-swathe. With it, you can treat a number of different upper body fractures.

Fractures of the upper arm bone, the humerus, can be adequately splinted in a sling-and-swathe without any stiff or rigid material. When the arm is secured to the chest wall with one or two swathes, the chest wall serves as part of the splint. Patients often feel more comfortable with their elbow out of the sling, allowing it to hang free and thus prevent upward pressure on the arm from the sling. Fractures of the collarbone (clavicle) are adequately treated with a sling-and-swathe that supports the full weight of the arm. Unlike

Upper Arm Fractures

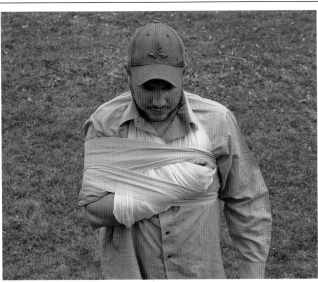

- Fractures of the upper arm bone can be splinted with a sling-and-swathe.

- There is no need to provide rigid support for the lower arm.

- Patients may feel less pain if the elbow hangs outside the sling, allowing gravity

to pull gentle traction on the fracture site.

- A swathe needs to hold the upper arm securely to the chest wall. Use a wide swathe to disperse pressure on the upper arm.

Elbow Fractures

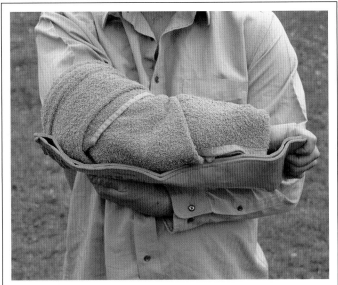

- Fractures in the region of the elbow can be splinted using a sling-and-swathe as the primary support.

- Place bulky padding around the elbow first. Apply the padding loosely to prevent discomfort to the patient.

- Secure a rigid support to the lower arm to provide additional security to the fracture site.

- After the arm is held in a sling, apply a wide swathe to hold the upper arm to the chest wall.

fractures of the humerus, clavicle fractures feel better when the weight of the arm is not pulling down on the shoulder. Fractures in the region of the elbow are best treated with a splint and a sling-and-swathe as described in "Splint a Lower Arm." Prior to attaching the splint, wrap the elbow well in soft material. With most fractures of the shoulder blade (scapula), a sling-and-swathe is adequate treatment.

A sling-and-swathe can also be used to stabilize the arm on the side of the chest that has suffered a fractured rib to ease pain and provide protection.

Clavicle Fractures

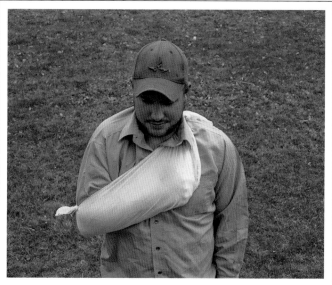

- Fractures of the collarbone can be adequately splinted with a properly applied sling-and-swathe.

- The sling needs to cup the elbow and hold it up to prevent gravity from pulling down on the broken bone.

- Secure the sling around the patient's neck in a way that does not press on the fractured bone.

- Apply a wide swathe to hold the upper arm to the chest wall, further preventing movement of the injury.

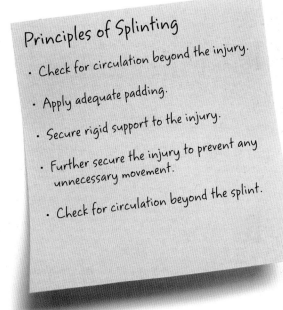

Principles of Splinting

- Check for circulation beyond the injury.

- Apply adequate padding.

- Secure rigid support to the injury.

- Further secure the injury to prevent any unnecessary movement.

- Check for circulation beyond the splint.

SPLINT A LEG
A good leg splint follows the same principles as a good arm splint

If you can splint an arm well, you can splint a leg well—the same principles are involved.

Fractures of the ankle require adequate padding with soft material around the ankle to avoid natural hollows and to provide comfort. The stiff or rigid material needs to maintain the foot at 90 degrees to the leg.

Fractures of the lower leg (tibia and/or fibula) require adequate padding around the ankle and behind the knee. The rigid material should be long enough to stabilize the ankle and the knee. If either joint moves, the fracture may shift.

Fractures in the region of the knee require adequate padding around the knee and stiff or rigid material to keep the knee from moving.

Fractures of the upper leg (femur) are typically among the most painful. The leg should be stabilized from hip to ankle, and the patient should be moved as gently as possible.

Ankle Fractures

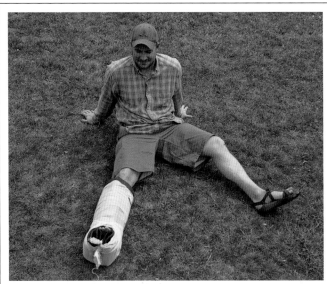

- The best splints for an ankle involve most of the lower leg.

- Wrap padding around the ankle and foot. The padding should extend up to at least the calf.

- Padding will provide comfort and protection and fill the natural voids around the ankle to further prevent movement.

- Secure rigid support to the lower leg. The rigid support should involve the foot in a manner that prevents flexion and extension of the foot.

Lower Leg Fractures

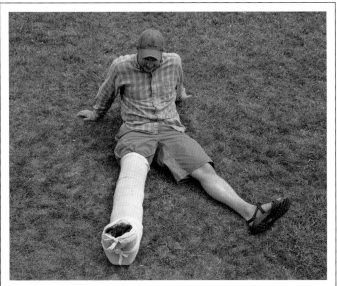

- The best splints for a lower leg fracture should restrict movement of the knee and ankle.

- The soft padding you apply around the leg should fill the natural voids around the knee and ankle.

- Place additional soft material behind the knee to keep the leg slightly flexed for comfort.

- The rigid support should be well secured above and below the knee, and it should prevent flexion and extension of the foot.

Fractures in the region of the hip can be adequately stabilized by padding between the patient's legs and securing the "bad" leg to the "good" leg.

Fractures of the pelvis are potentially the most devastating. Bleeding into the abdominal cavity is not uncommon. Gently tie a wide band of material around the pelvis, and move the patient only with great care.

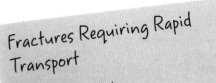

·············· RED ● LIGHT ··············

With any fracture you assess, if you find an open wound or exposed bone ends, rinse or irrigate the site thoroughly with clean water and apply a sterile dressing prior to splinting.

Upper Leg Fractures

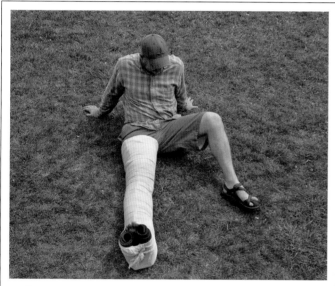

- The upper leg bone is a large bone with a large artery near it, and your care needs to be especially gentle.

- The best upper leg splints involve the entire leg with additional padding behind the knee for comfort.

- The patient should be kept as still as possible to prevent unnecessary movement of the hip.

- This fracture carries the potential for blood loss into the thigh, and an ambulance should be called as soon as possible.

Fractures Requiring Rapid Transport

- Exposed bone ends
- Open wound at fracture site
- Angulations caused by fracture
- Femur, hip, and pelvic fractures

DISLOCATIONS

Simple dislocations can sometimes be put back into place in an emergency

All dislocations carry the risk of inadequate circulation to the dislocated joint. In extreme circumstances, you may choose to attempt a reduction of the joint.

Finger dislocations are among the most common and often are reducible by a simple but gentle pull on the end of the dislocated finger. Hold the patient's hand in one of your hands, keep the finger flexed, and pull gently but steadily with your other hand in line with how the finger presents.

Kneecap (patella) dislocations will almost always reduce if you gently straighten the affected leg. If the patella does not immediately relocate, a gentle push on the side of the patella often completes the job.

Finger Dislocations 1

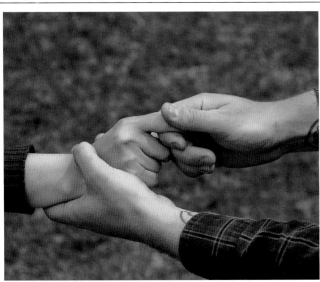

- Fingers most often dislocate at the middle joint, and that joint is the easiest to reduce.

- Hold the patient's hand in one of your hands, and take hold of the end of the dislocated finger with your other hand.

- Keep the patient's finger flexed and not straight.

- Pull in line with the way the finger presents. Pull steadily—do not jerk. Under your pressure, most finger joints will slide back into normal alignment.

Finger Dislocations 2

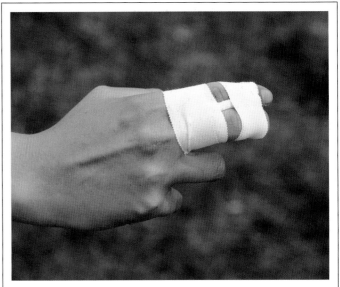

- Reduced or not, the joint is going to swell, and the application of ice is strongly recommended.

- Splint the finger by securing it to a healthy neighboring finger.

- Start by placing a pad of soft material between the two fingers, and then tape the two fingers together.

- Place strips of tape above and below the injured joint and not over the joint. The patient can now gently move the joint, and that will be beneficial.

70

Shoulder dislocations are more problematic, but a simple reduction method is often effective. Ask the patient to lie down. Then pull gentle, steady traction on the affected arm in line with how the patient presents, keeping the arm flexed and not straightened. Under traction, move the upper arm slowly away from the body, as if the patient was winding up to throw a ball.

All dislocations, reduced or not, need to be splinted.

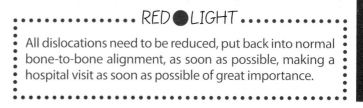

• • • • • • • • • • • • • • • *RED* ● *LIGHT* • • • • • • • • • • • • • • •

All dislocations need to be reduced, put back into normal bone-to-bone alignment, as soon as possible, making a hospital visit as soon as possible of great importance.

Kneecap Dislocations

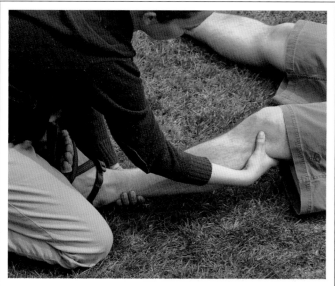

- Kneecaps can dislocate to the inside or the outside of the leg, but dislocations to the outside are far more common.

- There may be quite a bit of pain.

- To reduce, you must gently straighten the injured leg.

- This is usually best done by supporting the knee with one hand and straightening the leg from the ankle with your other hand.

- If the kneecap does not slide back into place, push it gently with the hand supporting the knee.

Shoulder Dislocations

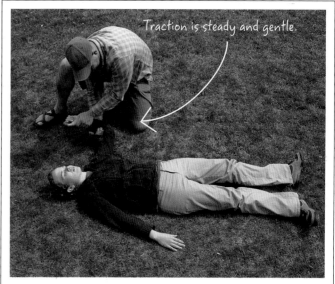

Traction is steady and gentle.

- It is best to start with the patient lying down. This technique may take several minutes.

- Position yourself at the patient's elbow and pull gently and steadily in line with the way the patient presents the arm on the injured side.

- If the shoulder remains unreduced, move the upper arm, still under your traction, externally, away from the body.

- If the shoulder remains unreduced, gently move the arm back to the body, and sling-and-swathe it.

71

BRUISES & SMALL CUTS
Proper treatment of small wounds prevents them from becoming big emergencies

Bruises, scrapes (see "Abrasions"), and small cuts comprise the vast majority of injuries to soft tissue. They are seldom serious, but proper management means the best outcome for the patient.

Bruises seldom require emergency care, but large bruises may benefit from cold, compression, and/or elevation. Substantial bruises should cause you to assess the patient for damage to underlying structures such as bones or organs such as the brain (see "Check the Head"), the lungs (see "Check the Chest"), and abdominal organs (see "Check the Abdomen").

Direct pressure on a small wound will stop the bleeding (see "Stop Bleeding 1"). The risk to the patient is the potential

Bruises

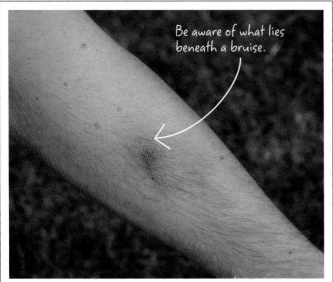

Be aware of what lies beneath a bruise.

- Bruises are extremely common and rarely serious.

- Deep and extensive bruising, however, can cause pain and swelling, and it can be treated with a cold pack and perhaps, depending on the body part, with compression from an elastic wrap.

- Bruising can also develop over a fracture site, and a patient with such bruising needs to be evaluated for a fracture.

- Be aware that deep bruising over a body cavity such as the chest or abdomen is an indication of the possibility of internal damage.

Step 1: Clean Small Wounds

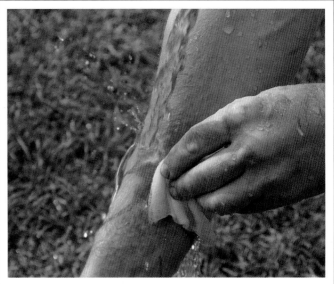

- The risk of infection exists with all wounds, no matter how small.

- Most small wound infections can be prevented with adequate cleaning.

- Irrigating the wound with running water is the best cleaning method. The

water can be from a tap or from an irrigation syringe included in some first-aid kits.

- Soap is not required, but, if you use soap, it needs to be irrigated from the wound after application.

for infection. Adequate wound cleaning, dressing, and bandaging will prevent most wound infections. Running water from a household faucet will adequately clean small wounds. Allow the water to run through the wound for about a minute.

Technically speaking, a dressing goes directly on the wound, and a bandage holds the dressing in place. Small, adhesive strip bandages are both dressing and bandage. Larger combination dressings and bandages are available and make great additions to your first-aid kit.

············· GREEN ● LIGHT ··············

Tetanus, a serious infection possible with many wounds, can be prevented with a vaccination. The vaccination must be updated at least every ten years. Ask your patient about his or her vaccination status.

Step 2: Dress the Wound

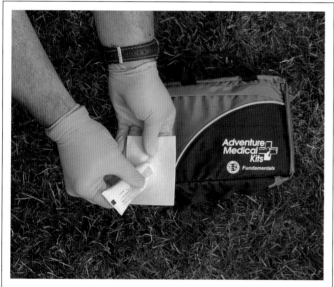

- A dressing is the material placed directly onto a clean wound.

- A dressing needs to be sterile, which means, in most cases, it is material sterilized during the manufacturing process and sealed in a closed packet.

- Some dressings are made with a surface that prevents the material from sticking to the wound, making removal easy and painless.

- If the dressing you use is not nonsticking, consider applying an antibiotic ointment prior to applying it.

Step 3: Bandage the Wound

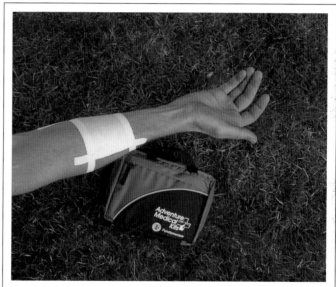

- The bandage is the material used to hold the dressing in place.

- All first-aid kits and almost all homes have adhesive strip bandages that are actually a combination of a dressing and a bandage.

- Bandaging material that is not adhesive can be held in place with tape or an elastic wrap.

- The dressing and bandage should be changed daily, allowing for inspection of the wound for signs of infection.

DEEP CUTS

Deep cuts, in an emergency, can sometimes be managed without stitches

Most deep cuts—those that penetrate the full thickness of the skin and enter the muscle beneath—should be closed by a physician. There may be, however, situations where a physician is not readily available, and you may choose to close a deep cut.

Before closure, cuts (lacerations) require aggressive clean-ing. This should be done via irrigation. Irrigation syringes are included in many high-quality first-aid kits. The pressure from most household faucets is adequate for cleaning. Irrigation should use at least a half-liter of water from a syringe or at least a minute of irrigation from a faucet.

Dry the skin with sterile gauze. Then cuts can be closed

Step 1: Clean

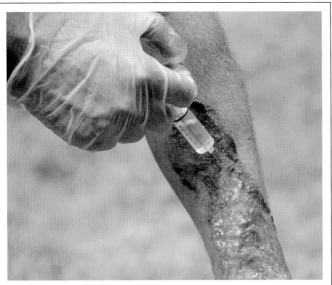

- The deeper the wound, the more important the job of cleaning becomes.

- There is no great rush. Be sure that you have stopped the bleeding and that the torn vessels have had time to fully clot.

- Before cleaning the wound itself, wash around the wound with soap and water, and rinse the area thoroughly.

- Be sure to hold the wound open during irrigation in order to clean all the way to the bottom.

Step 2: Close

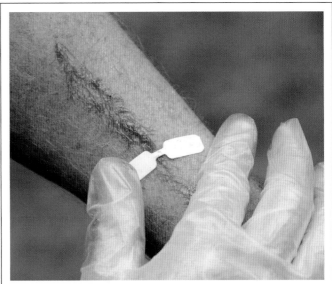

- Do not attempt to suture or staple a wound closed at home. These procedures should be performed by a physician.

- Use wound closure strips, or cut tape into thin strips.

- Tape the edges of the wound back in their original position as precisely as possible—not too tight, not too loose.

- The application of tincture of benzoin compound near the wound's edges prior to closure will make the closure strips stick better.

with "butterfly" adhesive strips or, even better, with skin closure strips. A thin coat of tincture of benzoin compound applied to the skin around the wound prior to the strips aids in adhesion of the strips. Benzoin is an irritant, so take care to keep it out of the wound. Let the benzoin dry for at least thirty seconds before applying the strips. The closure strips may be applied perpendicular to the wound. Apply one to one side of the wound and another to the opposite side. By using the opposing strips as handles, you can pull the wound edges together, pulling the skin as close as possible to where

it should lie naturally but without pulling the wound tightly shut. In the absence of butterfly strips or closure strips, wound closure may be accomplished with thin strips of whatever tape happens to be available. The wound should be covered with sterile bandaging material. Small, deep wounds cleaned and closed properly with adhesive strips have a very low incidence of infection, but the wound requires a daily check for signs of infection: increasing pain, redness, swelling, and perhaps pus.

Step 3: Dress and Bandage

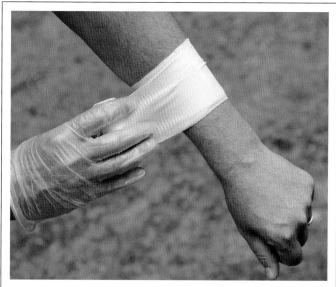

- As with small wounds, the injury needs to be appropriately dressed and bandaged.

- The dressing needs to extend about one-half inch beyond the ends of the closure strips. If the ends of the strips are visible, germs can migrate along the strips to reach the wound.

- Consider adding microthin film dressings to your first-aid kit. They are germ barriers that you can see through, allowing you to monitor the wound.

- Do not use antibiotic ointment underneath microthin dressings.

Symptoms of Wound Infection

- Redness extending more than one-quarter inch from the wound

- Unusual warmth at the wound site

- Increasing swelling

- Increasing pain

- Pus

ABRASIONS

Abrasions can be painful but are seldom serious unless they get infected

When skin is scraped (abraded) away, the shallow wound is an abrasion. Abrasions are common and rarely serious—unless they get infected.

Abrasions are an exception to the rule of wound cleaning: You need to scrub the surface of the wound to achieve adequate cleaning. A sterile gauze pad is adequate for scrubbing.

Scrubbing may be enhanced by using any soap, but all soap should be carefully rinsed and then irrigated from the wound after scrubbing. It is important to remove all embedded debris not only to reduce the risk of infection but also to prevent subsequent "tattooing" (scarring) of the skin. With a deep abrasion, self-scrubbing is seldom successful due to

Step 1: Scrub

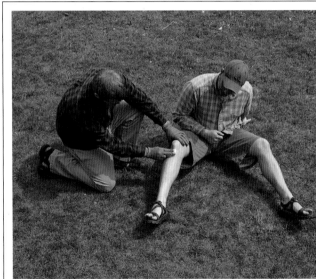

- Abrasions have a relatively high rate of infection due to the fact that germs are often deeply embedded in the wound when the injury occurs.

- Abrasions, therefore, should be scrubbed clean with soft material and soap and water.

- The scrubbing process can be painful for the patient. You need to scrub gently but firmly.

- After the abrasion has been thoroughly scrubbed, the soap needs to be rinsed, flushed, or irrigated out of the wound.

Step 2: Dress

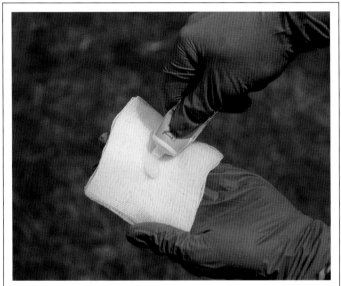

- If abrasions are allowed to completely dry, a scab will form.

- Scabs are not harmful, but a scab-covered wound will take longer to heal, and the chance of a scar forming is greater.

- To prevent scab formation, cover an abrasion liberally with an antibiotic ointment prior to applying a dressing. It is best to apply the ointment to the dressing, then the dressing to the wound.

- The ointment will also prevent the dressing from sticking to the wound.

the high level of pain associated with the exposed nerves.

After cleansing, prevent the surface of abrasions from drying out (but not with water). Drying causes scab formation, which is not bad but increases healing time. Apply a topical agent, such as an antibiotic ointment, followed by a dressing of a sterile gauze pad or a roll of sterile gauze to keep the ointment in place. Tape may be used to hold a sterile gauze pad in place. Commercial dressings are available to cover abrasions. Ideally, dressings should be changed twice a day and/or any time the dressing gets wet.

Step 3: Bandage

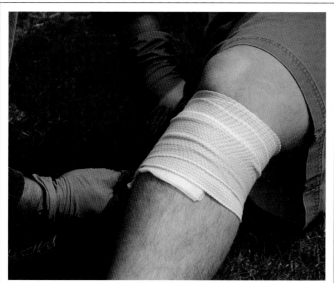

- In fact, an abrasion covered in antibiotic ointment is dressed, and there is no medical reason for anything else.

- But the ointment gets rubbed off, and this presents the need for a means to keep it in place.

- The additional dressing material, such as a gauze pad, will hold the antibiotic, but you still need a bandage to hold the gauze in place.

- You can use tape, an elastic wrap, or a length of roller gauze to do the job.

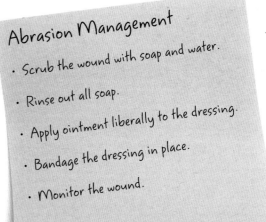

Abrasion Management

- Scrub the wound with soap and water.

- Rinse out all soap.

- Apply ointment liberally to the dressing.

- Bandage the dressing in place.

- Monitor the wound.

AMPUTATIONS

Amputations almost always result in the loss of the body part—but not always

When a body part is torn or cut completely off, you have an amputation. (If a piece of skin is partially cut off, it is often called an "avulsion.") With proper care, the amputated part can sometimes be reattached.

The first concern of the first-aid provider is stopping serious bleeding (see "Stop Bleeding"). Do not attempt to reattach the body part. If a detached body part can be easily recovered, and if the patient can be brought to a hospital within six hours, even longer for fingers and toes, reattachment may be possible. The body part should be quickly flushed with clean water to remove contaminants. The part should then be wrapped in slightly moistened sterile gauze and placed in

Step 1: Treat the Patient

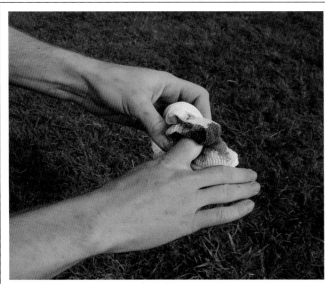

- Your immediate concern with a patient who has an amputated body part is stopping the flow of blood from the patient.

- This often requires less attention to the wound than you might think.

- Cleanly amputated parts typically allow the blood vessels in the area to retract into the patient, causing less blood loss than if they did not retract.

- Direct pressure on the wound is usually all that is required.

Step 2: Treat the Part

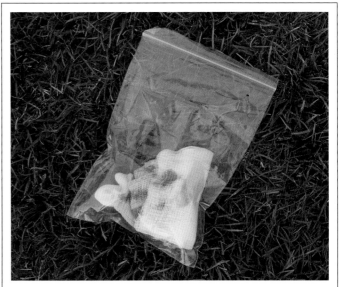

- As soon as possible, recover the amputated part, and rinse it gently clean with the cleanest water available. Do not scrub the part.

- Wet and wring the excess water from a sterile gauze pad. If you do not have sterile gauze, use the cleanest material available.

- Wrap the amputated part in the damp material, and seal the part in a plastic bag.

- The dampness will prevent the amputated part from drying out, improving the chance that it can be reattached.

a plastic bag. Keep the part cold with a cold pack or with ice, if available. Or place the plastic bag containing the body part in a water bottle filled with the coldest water possible. Do not apply ice directly to the body part or else frostbite may ensue, and do not place the part directly in water.

The wound on the patient should then be irrigated and bandaged. (An avulsion should be cleaned and, if transport is delayed, taped to hold it in its natural position and covered with a sterile dressing.)

Step 3: Chill the Part

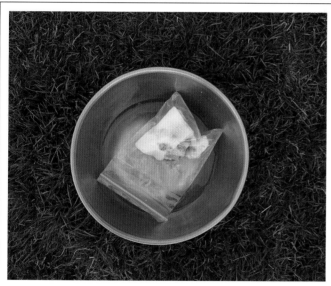

- The amputated part will have the best chance of reattachment if it is also kept cool. It cannot, however, be frozen.

- Once in a plastic bag, it can be placed on ice or on a cold pack.

- It can also be placed in ice water or the coldest water available.

- The faster the transport of the patient and the amputated part to a hospital, the greater the chance of reattachment.

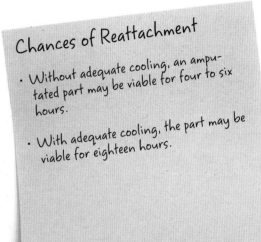

Chances of Reattachment

- Without adequate cooling, an amputated part may be viable for four to six hours.

- With adequate cooling, the part may be viable for eighteen hours.

IMPALEMENTS

In most cases, if something is embedded in a patient, it should stay there

Large objects found impaled in a wound should be left in place in almost all cases. Attempting to remove an object can stimulate serious bleeding and damage underlying structures, especially if the object is impaled in a body cavity, that is, chest, abdomen, or head. The object should be stabilized with padding to prevent movement. The padding

should be as high as the object, if possible, to protect it from being bumped during transport, and the patient should be carried.

In some instances, an impaled object makes movement of the patient difficult. The object may be extremely large, or the patient may be impaled on an unmovable object. In

Impalement

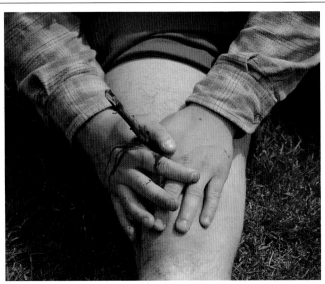

- When an object is impaled into a patient's body, damage is done during the entry.

- There is also an excellent chance that more damage will be done when the object is removed.

- Any movement of the object while it is impaled can cause damage to the tissues into which the object is impaled.

- In almost all cases, an impaled object should be left in place and moved as little as possible.

Padding

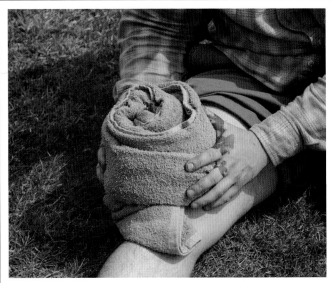

- Typically, there is little blood loss around an impaled object because the object is wedged tightly into the wound.

- Thick, clean padding—any soft material—should be carefully placed around the impaled object. Do this without moving the object.

- If possible, the padding should reach all the way to the top of the object.

- The purpose of the padding is to secure the object as it lies, preventing any further movement.

these instances, you must find professional help as soon as possible.

If the object is impaled through a cheek or in any other way endangering the patient's airway, there is general agreement among experts that the object should be carefully removed, if possible.

Objects impaled in the eye should never be removed. A patient with an impaled object in the eye should have the object well protected against movement, both eyes should be covered, and the patient should be carried.

Secure the Padding

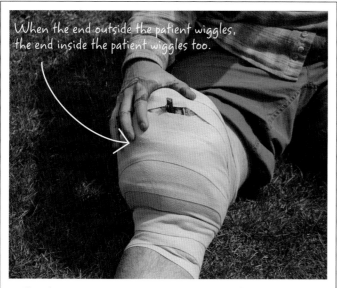

When the end outside the patient wiggles, the end inside the patient wiggles too.

- The object is not secured in place until the padding has been secured in place.

- You can do this with elastic wraps or with strips of soft material. You can use tape, but tear off strips of tape before applying them to the patient.

- While securing the padding in place, move the patient, and therefore the object, as little as possible.

- If possible, do not move the patient. Call for help, and wait until professional assistance arrives to transport the patient.

Impalement Management

- Do not attempt to remove the object.

- Avoid any unnecessary movement of the patient or the object.

- Place thick, clean padding around the object.

- Secure the padding in place.

- Call for help!

BURNS

Burns range from a relatively mild discomfort to a threat to life

Large burns are among the most painful and emotionally distressing of injuries. Although burns may result from electricity, radiation, and chemicals, burns treated by first-aid providers most often result from high heat sources: (1) scalding hot water, (2) open flames, or (3) hot objects. In all cases, immediate first aid is critically important.

If necessary, remove the patient from the source of the burn.

Stop the burning process. The faster, the better, within thirty seconds if possible. Burns can continue to injure tissue for a surprisingly long time after the source of the burn is removed. Smother flames, if appropriate, and then *cool the burn with cool water*. There are also several commercial products, such as burn gels and burn dressings, appropriate for application immediately to a burn site. In general, cooling should continue as long as the patient is experiencing pain.

Cool the Burn

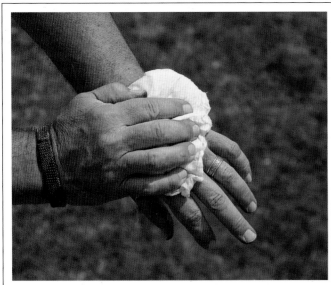

- Just as a stick keeps burning after removal from a fire, a body part keeps burning after removal from the source of the burn.

- To stop the burning process, apply cold water to the burn site. Do this immediately!

- The burn site can be placed in cold water, or a soaking wet compress can be placed on the burn site.

- Continue the cooling process until the patient denies pain.

Swelling

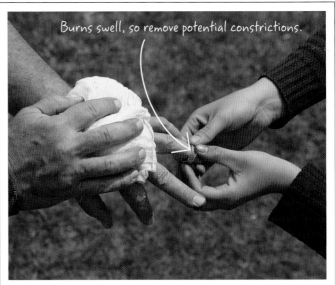

Burns swell, so remove potential constrictions.

- A burn injury will swell. Constrictions in the area of a burn can cut off circulation, causing further harm.

- Remove clothing from a burn site, and remove anything that could become a constriction, such as rings, watches, and jewelry.

- But do *not* attempt to remove synthetic clothing that has melted into the burn site.

- Burns that entirely encircle an extremity can swell to the point where the burn itself cuts off circulation. These burns require rapid access to transportation.

Remove clothing and jewelry from the burn area. Do not try to remove tar or melted plastic, including synthetic clothing, if it is stuck to the burn.

Cover cooled burns with clean, soft material. If blisters develop, attempt to prevent them from popping open.

·········· RED ● LIGHT ···········

It is difficult to evaluate the damage a burn has done until time has passed. For that reason, large burns require a physician's care as soon as possible.

Burn Dressings

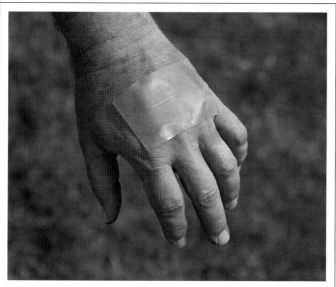

- Some burn dressings hold moisture in a gelatinous form and continue the cooling process after being applied.

- These dressings may be in the form of burn gels or burn sheets.

- If you have no burn dressings in your first-aid kit, cool the burn thoroughly, and then cover the burn site with clean, dry clothing.

- If blisters form, try to protect them from rupturing until you can find professional care.

Serious Burns

- Burns to the patient's airway

- Burns through the full thickness of the skin

- Large burns to face, hands, feet, armpits, and groin

- Burns that cover more than 10 percent of the patient's body

- Burns that entirely encompass an extremity

ANGINA

Angina is a condition that must be diagnosed by a physician

Pain caused by an interruption in an adequate flow of blood to the heart muscle is called *angina pectoris* (pain in the chest), but it is typically called simply *angina*. It is the result of cardiovascular disease that has created a narrowing of arteries that carry blood to the heart. Pain usually arrives on the heels of physical or emotional stress, events that increase the workload on the heart, but it can occur without stress.

The chest pain is most often sudden, and it can range from a mild ache to crushing pressure described as "squeezing," "tightness," "constricting," or sometimes "burning." It often radiates to the left shoulder and arm and less often to the neck, back, and/or jaw. And it may be accompanied by shortness of breath and nausea.

If this is not the first attack, a doctor may have prescribed nitroglycerin. It may be in the form of tablets or spray, and usually they both go under the tongue. If nitro is prescribed

Symptoms of Angina

- Persistent chest pain
- Shortness of breath
- Dizziness or light-headedness
- Pale, cool, sweaty skin
- Nausea, perhaps vomiting
- Fast, slow, weak, and/or irregular heartbeat

Treatment

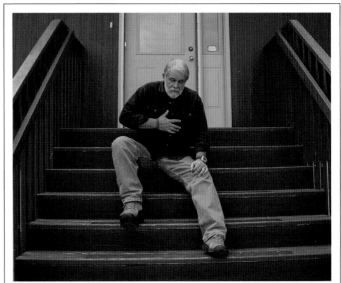

- Keep the patient physically and emotionally calm. Speak in a calm and reassuring voice.

- Aid the patient in assuming a position that provides the most comfort, but ideally do not allow the patient to walk.

- Protect the patient from loss of body heat with a blanket or other insulating material.

- If it is angina, the attack will pass with rest and/or medication. But do not leave the patient unattended.

and available, help the patient take it. If the pain persists ten minutes later, help the patient take a second dose. Three doses in all may be taken.

Nitroglycerin

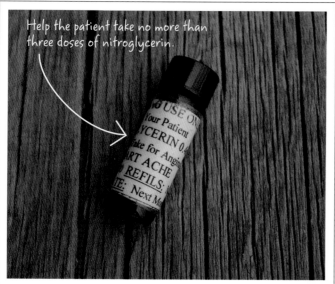

Help the patient take no more than three doses of nitroglycerin.

- Nitroglycerin is the drug prescribed for patients diagnosed with angina.

- It is often a small white pill placed under the tongue. Nitro stings when placed under the tongue, a sign that the drug is working.

- You should find a strong pulse at the wrist before helping someone take nitro.

- If transportation is not readily available, a second pill may be taken after ten minutes if pain persists. A third pill may be taken after another ten minutes.

Aspirin

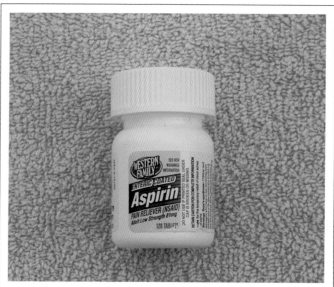

- Aspirin is recommended for patients suffering an attack of angina unless they have received different instructions prior to their attack.

- The recommended dose is one adult aspirin (325 milligrams) or four "baby" aspirins (81 milligrams each).

- Aspirin will act more quickly if the tablets are chewed and quickly swallowed, but simple swallowing is acceptable.

- If transportation is severely delayed, the dose of aspirin should be repeated every twenty-four hours until a physician's care is available.

HEART ATTACK

Heart attacks remain the number one killers of people in the United States

A heart attack, or myocardial infarction (MI), occurs when a clot completely blocks or reduces the blood flow through an artery carrying blood to the heart muscle to the point that the part of the heart fed by that artery dies. If the part of the heart is large, the heart stops.

Although a heart attack can be painless, it will most often resemble an attack of angina (see "Angina"), with crushing, squeezing chest pain or "heavy pressure" in the chest that may radiate to the left shoulder and arm, perhaps to the jaw and back. The patient's pulse will probably be weak, maybe rapid, or sometimes slow and regular or irregular in rhythm. Rapid, shallow breathing is common, as is the complaint of

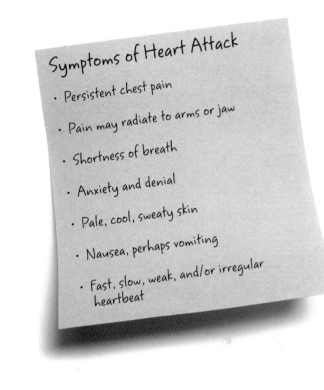

Symptoms of Heart Attack

- Persistent chest pain
- Pain may radiate to arms or jaw
- Shortness of breath
- Anxiety and denial
- Pale, cool, sweaty skin
- Nausea, perhaps vomiting
- Fast, slow, weak, and/or irregular heartbeat

Treatment 1

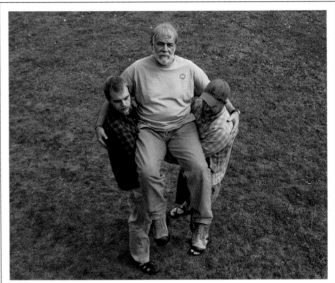

- Keep the patient physically and emotionally calm. Speak in a calm and reassuring voice.

- If in doubt, assume it is a heart attack. Patients so often deny a heart attack that "denial" is considered a sign.

- Do not allow the patient to exercise. Exercise can make the attack worse. If the patient must be moved, carry the patient even short distances.

- As soon as possible call or send someone to call 911.

shortness of breath. The patient's skin is usually pale, cool, and sweaty. And surprisingly common is the fact that the patient may deny the possibility that this could be a heart attack.

The patient must be kept physically and emotionally calm, in the position that feels most comfortable, and protected against loss of body heat.

If aspirin is available, it should be offered to the patient, one adult aspirin or four children's aspirins. In both cases, the aspirin will get to work faster if chewed before swallowing.

Treatment 2

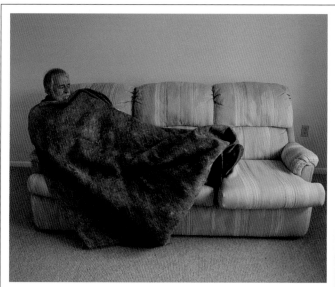

- Aid the patient in assuming a position that provides the most comfort. This position is often a semireclining position.

- Protect the patient from loss of body heat with a blanket or other insulating material.

- Unless otherwise instructed, give the patient one adult aspirin (325 milligrams) or four "baby" aspirins (81 milligrams each).

- If it is a heart attack, it is unlikely that the attack will pass. In all cases, do not leave the patient unattended.

All victims of heart attack need to be cared for at a hospital as soon as possible. They should never walk because even mild exertion could greatly exacerbate the problem.

Cardiac Emergency Management

- Keep the patient physically and emotionally calm.

- Allow no exercise.

- Help the patient find a position of comfort.

- Protect from loss of body heat.

- Give aspirin.

- Call 911.

CARDIAC & RESPIRATORY

87

HYPERVENTILATION

When someone is breathing much faster than normal, it could be a simple problem

As a first-aid provider, you will encounter little that is more important than making sure your patient keeps breathing. Some of your patients, however, will breathe faster and/or more deeply than normal, a syndrome called *hyperventilation*. Hyperventilation can be voluntary, but it often has a cause that could be minor or could be serious. You need to

figure out which—and treat it appropriately.

Hyperventilation is a response to some type of stress, real or imagined, and a high level of anxiety or panic is common. It often causes numbness or tingling in the hands, feet, and mouth. There may be muscular spasms in the hands and feet. A feeling of tightness in the chest is also common, as are

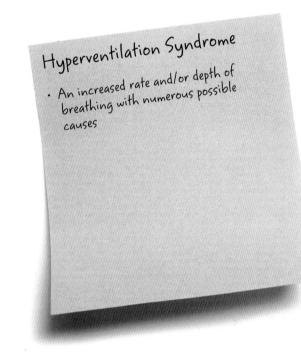

Hyperventilation Syndrome

- An increased rate and/or depth of breathing with numerous possible causes

Reassurance

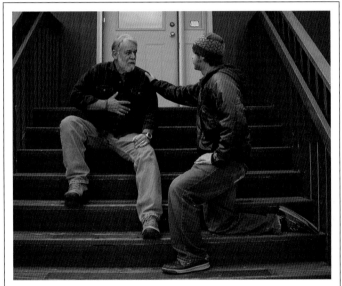

- Rapidly assess the patient to determine the cause of hyperventilation, and treat causes if found.

- Hyperventilation syndrome is usually brought on by anxiety, but it can be produced by pain, and it can be voluntary.

- Patients often feel like they are suffocating. They may be feeling chest pain and tingling or numbness in hands, feet, or face.

- Make eye contact, speak directly but reassuringly, and tell patients they are able to and need to regain control of their breathing.

complaints of light-headedness or dizziness. These feelings do *not* help the patient calm down.

Prolonged hyperventilation may lead to fainting. After fainting, the patient may not breathe for an alarming number of seconds. But the patient will resume breathing if there is no life-threatening cause.

A life-threatening cause, such as a hole in the chest, should be immediately treated. An emotionally stressful cause, such as a high school prom, requires calming reassurance by the rescuer. In any case, remember to stay calm.

······· GREEN ● LIGHT ·············

Patients who are hyperventilating without a medically serious cause will eventually calm down and resume normal breathing. Their recovery will be complete and typically not more than twenty to thirty minutes away.

Breathing Control

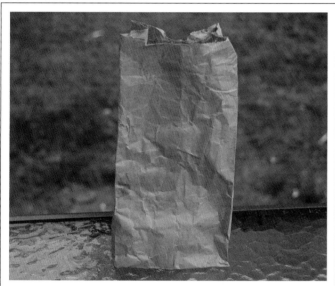

- Breathing into a paper bag has a long history but is now recognized as counterproductive. Forget the paper bag.

- Tell patients they are feeling the physical symptoms due to the way they are breathing.

- In a firm but reassuring voice, tell patients to breathe with you, and demonstrate slow breaths with obvious pauses between breaths.

- In extreme cases, the patient will pass out. Position the patient on a side. Breathing will resume.

Hyperventilation Management

- Calm the patient.

- Make eye contact.

- Speak firmly but reassuringly.

- Encourage the patient to breathe slowly.

CARDIAC & RESPIRATORY

89

ASTHMA

Attacks of this chronic disease range from mild to life-threatening

An asthma attack involves swelling of the airway, increased production of sticky mucus in the airway, and spasms of the airway, all of which cause difficulty breathing. Your intervention, if needed, can have life-saving results.

Patients suffering mild asthma typically deal with it by exerting self-control of breathing and/or inhaling medication from an over-the-counter inhaler.

Moderate asthma sufferers usually carry a prescription-strength medication, often inhaled through a spacer, a tube connected to the inhaler that captures and concentrates the drug inhaled. Sometimes these inhaled drugs are for prevention, and sometimes they are prescribed for an acute attack.

Severe asthmatics may be taking an oral drug to help control their disease, and these individuals are the most susceptible to a severe attack.

If you are involved, you should calmly encourage the patient

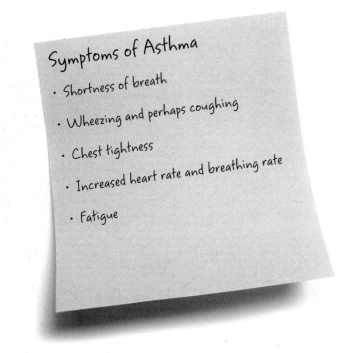

Symptoms of Asthma

- Shortness of breath
- Wheezing and perhaps coughing
- Chest tightness
- Increased heart rate and breathing rate
- Fatigue

Inhalers

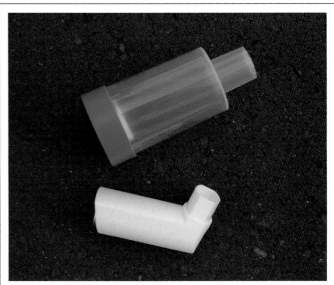

- Over-the-counter inhalers are available (without a prescription) for sufferers of mild asthma.

- Stronger medications (often albuterol) are prescribed for people who suffer more serious attacks, and these drugs, too, are carried in inhalers.

- These drugs are bronchodilaters. They open up (dilate) the narrowed air passages of the patient.

- The drugs are delivered from the inhaler as a mist that must be inhaled deeply to be effective.

to relax and breathe with control. The patient may need help finding and using the inhaler. The inhaler should be held with the mouthpiece on the bottom, shaken, and placed with the mouthpiece between the lips. The patient should exhale prior to pressing the container into the mouthpiece, releasing the misted drug, which is then inhaled as deeply as possible.

Patients who are having difficulty exhaling may be encouraged to exhale against pursed lips, sort of like blowing out a candle.

A mild asthma attack does not require the care of a physician, but monitor the patient, watching for a relapse. A severe attack should be immediately evaluated by a physician.

Inhaling the Drug

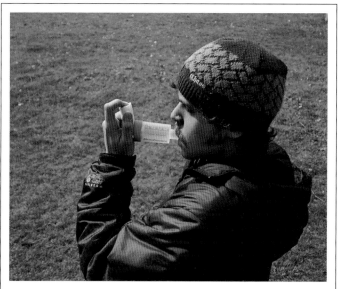

After Inhaling

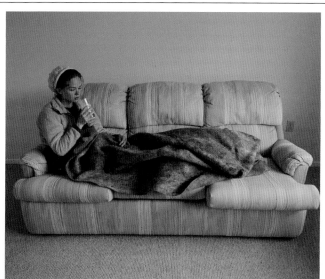

CARDIAC & RESPIRATORY

- Many asthma sufferers carry a spacer, a tube connected to the port of the inhaler.

- A spacer captures the misted drug, allowing more of the drug to be inhaled for greater effectiveness.

- The inhaler should be held with the port down and then shaken before delivery of the drug. The patient needs to exhale before depressing the inhaler to release the drug.

- The usual dose is two puffs every five minutes up to twelve puffs until the attack ends.

- An asthma attack is fatiguing, and the patient should be encouraged to rest in a comfortable position until normal activity can be resumed.

- The patient may be thirsty and may be encouraged to drink water.

- Patients who state that the attack is their worst or equal to their worst should be evaluated by a physician. Speed is not required.

- Patients who do not respond to their medication require rapid transport to a hospital.

PNEUMONIA

Pneumonia causes an accumulation of fluid in the lungs that can be fatal

Pneumonia is an infection in the lungs caused by a wide variety of agents, including bacteria, viruses, protozoa, and fungi. The disease process can cause swelling and fluid collection in the lungs, leading to difficulty breathing. Pneumonia is, far more often than not, curable. Unfortunately and despite antibiotic therapy, it will still be the fifth or sixth leading cause of death in the United States this year.

A patient most in need of emergency care will probably have an infection, most likely bacterial, which produces any or all of six classic signs and symptoms: shortness of breath (the most important), chest pain, chills, fever, increased sputum production, and a productive cough—a cough that may produce

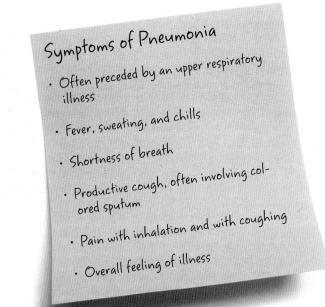

Symptoms of Pneumonia

- Often preceded by an upper respiratory illness
- Fever, sweating, and chills
- Shortness of breath
- Productive cough, often involving colored sputum
- Pain with inhalation and with coughing
- Overall feeling of illness

Maintaining an Airway

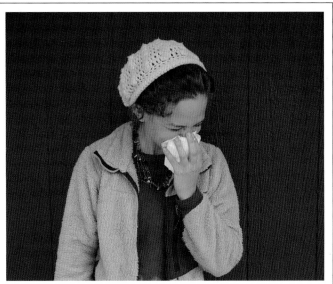

- With pneumonia, the air passages swell, and mucus production increases, making breathing problematic. You may hear wet breath sounds when the patient breathes.

- Despite the fact that coughing often causes pain, the patient should be encour-aged to cough, bringing up the mucus and helping keep the air passages open.

- The patient should also be encouraged to breathe deeply to improve oxygenation.

- Supplemental oxygen would be of benefit to this patient.

sputum interestingly colored from yellowish to greenish, even brownish. The patient is typically "sick" and exhausted.

Pneumonia has a range of seriousness from mild to severe, but almost all cases require specific antibiotic treatment. The patient should be speedily transported to definitive medical care, preferably while breathing a high flow of supplemental oxygen. The patient may also be given antipyretic (antifever) drugs and should be kept well hydrated. Encourage the patient to breathe deeply from time to time and to cough up the sputum collecting in his or her upper airway.

Supportive Care

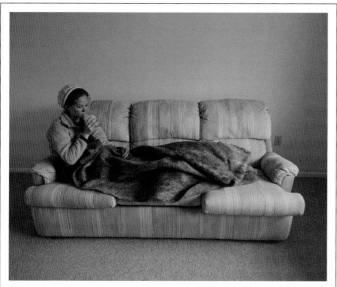

- A patient with pneumonia requires supportive care that encourages the healing process.

- Rest is extremely important, and patients should be allowed to choose the position, usually semireclining, that makes it easiest for them to breathe.

- Protection from loss of body heat during chills is mandatory.

- Adequate hydration is also mandatory. Fluids support the immune system and may help keep accumulating mucus mobile.

Medication

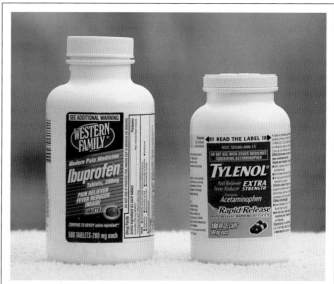

- Patients with pneumonia will benefit from fever-reducing drugs such as acetaminophen and ibuprofen.

- These drugs are available over the counter and should be given following the directions on the labels.

- Most cases of pneumonia,

however, require antibiotic therapy, and a physician should be consulted as soon as possible after pneumonia is suspected.

- Even with modern medications, pneumonia remains among the leading causes of death from illness in the United States.

FLULIKE ILLNESSES
Cold or flu? It's really the severity that dictates what you do

Flulike illnesses are often viral (although they can be bacterial) and are an infection of the nasal passages, throat, and sometimes the bronchi—and are thus sometimes referred to as "upper respiratory infections." Patients often complain that they have a "cold" but that this one is worse than usual. Flulike illnesses are often not serious.

Signs and symptoms may include increased mucus production (with the accompanying "runny nose"), sneezing, coughing that may be productive, sore throat, headache, muscle aches, a "run down" feeling, and a low fever. (If the problem is "stomach flu," there will be gastrointestinal signs and symptoms: nausea, vomiting, diarrhea.)

Patients need rest and hydration. Decongestants may be given for congestion, and acetaminophen or ibuprofen will work against the aches and fever. Although flulike illnesses are usually self-limiting, they can linger for weeks despite

Symptoms of Flulike Illnesses

- Headache

- Fever

- Muscle aches

- Nasal congestion and coughing

- General feelings of illness

Medications

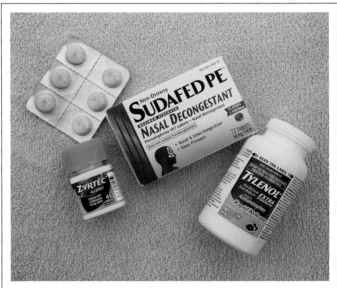

- Over-the-counter medications for the pain of headache and muscle aches include acetaminophen, aspirin, and ibuprofen. These same drugs will also help to reduce a fever.

- Over-the-counter medications for congestion, such as pseudoephedrine, may

be considered for adults.

- Over-the-counter antihistamines may be considered for runny noses.

- All these medications must be used only following the directions on the labels unless otherwise directed by a physician.

your best efforts at treatment. Patients who improve with treatment almost never require more than "home care."

Indicators that the patient could be seriously ill include a high fever—more than 102 degrees Fahrenheit (102°F)—headaches that don't respond to treatment, a stiff neck, inability to tolerate oral fluids (the patient throws up frequently), a sore throat that makes it difficult to swallow, a sore throat that makes the throat red with white patches, and the signs and symptoms of pneumonia (see "Pneumonia").

·············· RED ● LIGHT ··············

Patients who continue to deteriorate, despite your care, are more seriously ill and may need antibiotic therapy—and these patients should be evaluated by a physician.

Supportive Care

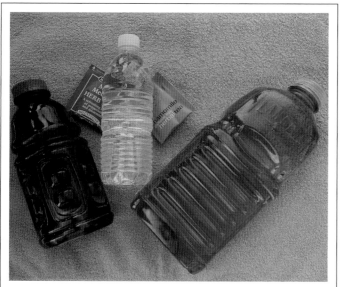

- Patients with flulike illnesses require supportive care to encourage the healing process.

- Adequate rest is important and should be continued until the signs and symptoms abate unless otherwise directed by a physician.

- Adequate hydration is critical. The patient should drink clear fluids that include but are not limited to water, herbal teas, clear fruit juices, broths, and perhaps sports drinks.

- Enough fluid should be consumed to maintain clear urine.

Danger!

- A high fever (102°F or more) that persists

- Severe headache unrelieved by medication and/or a stiff neck

- Wheezing and/or difficulty breathing

- Signs and symptoms of pneumonia

- Persistent vomiting and/or diarrhea

CARDIAC & RESPIRATORY

UNCONSCIOUS PATIENTS
Numerous causes can make a patient unresponsive

"Unconsciousness" can mean many things. On one end of the spectrum is the patient who is simply daydreaming, unaware of the immediate happenings, and on the other end is the completely unresponsive patient. You need to determine the level of responsiveness with all your patients. Unconscious patients may respond when you shout or when you stimulate them with pain, such as a pinch on the back of the arm. Or they might not respond at all.

The immediate emergency care, however, for all unconscious patients, despite the cause, is generally the same: (1) Protect the airway. Consider rolling the patient into the recovery position (to help maintain the airway). (2) Protect the spine unless you do not need to take spinal precautions (see "Check the Spine 1"). (3) Check thoroughly for a reason for the unconsciousness. Check carefully for medical alert tags. Check the pockets of the clothing for clues. Check purses

Recovery Position

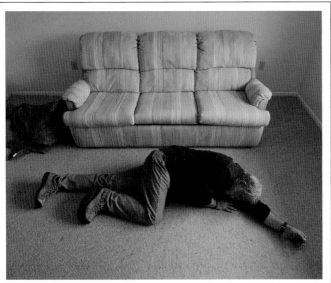

- Patients who are deeply unconscious and who are on their backs are at greater risk than patients on their sides.

- They lose control of their tongue, allowing the tongue to fall back and block the airway.

- If this patient vomits, the vomit may be inhaled into the lungs, with the likelihood of devastating results.

- For these reasons, the unconscious patient should be positioned in a stable side position, the recovery position (pictured).

Look for Clues 1

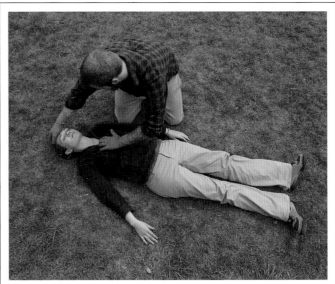

- You must sometimes be clever in your search for clues explaining the patient's unconsciousness.

- Look for damage to the head—bumps, bruises, cuts, depressions— evidence of trauma that could be the cause of unconsciousness.

- Check around the patient for clues: empty bottles, containers of anything that could have been ingested, partially eaten substances that could be the cause.

- Check the patient closely for additional clues: signs of incontinence, hidden wounds, unexplained marks.

and wallets. Ask bystanders who may know the patient. Look for clues near the patient, such as empty bottles or partially eaten substances. (4) Protect the patient from further harm.

Specific treatment will depend on the cause of unconsciousness, but consider giving sugar to patients unconscious for unknown reasons (see "Diabetes: Hypoglycemia").

Look for Clues 2

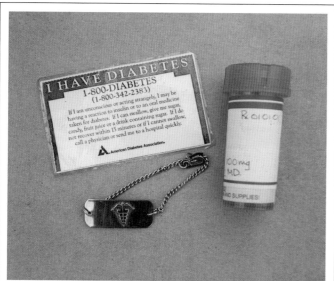

- Carefully check the patient's body for medical alert tags that could be worn at the neck, the wrist, or the ankle.

- Check the pockets, the wallet, the pocketbook, the backpack, the briefcase for medical alert cards or containers of drugs.

- Check the cell phone for a medical alert application that would explain underlying conditions the patient suffers.

- These types of clues can be the most valuable in determining what to do.

What Causes the Brain to Stop?

- Toxins, such as alcohol

- Seizure, stroke, or lack of sugar (diabetes)

- Temperature changes: too hot or too cold

- Lack of oxygen, as in suffocation

- Pressure increase from trauma to the head

NEUROLOGICAL & DIABETIC

STROKE

Signs and symptoms vary depending on the part of the brain affected

A stroke—also called a "cerebrovascular accident" (CVA)—is an interruption of normal blood flow to a part of the brain. The interruption could be caused by a blood clot forming in a cerebral artery, an embolus circulating into the brain from another part of the body to form a clot, or a hemorrhage from a cerebral artery. Similar to a heart attack, a stroke may be called a "brain attack." As a rescuer, you won't know the type of stroke, but you don't need to: The signs and symptoms are similar, as is the treatment.

Alterations in mental status are common—often described by ambiguous terms such as "confused," "stuporous," "semiconscious," "unconscious"—and may leave the patient unable

The Stroke Patient

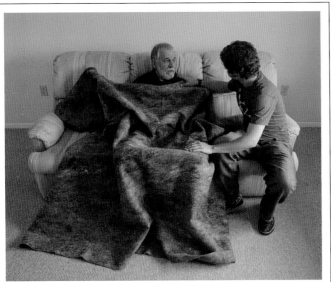

- A stroke can be similar to a heart attack, but it occurs in the brain.

- The patient typically experiences memory loss and appears dazed and confused. Weakness or paralysis may affect one side of the body, and facial paralysis may occur.

- The patient may be fully conscious but unable to speak or communicate in any way.

- The patient must be placed in a position of comfort, calmed and reassured, and not left unattended.

Recovery Position

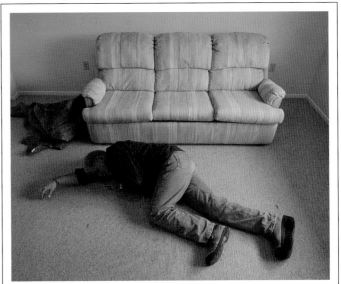

- If the stroke patient lapses into unconsciousness before the ambulance arrives, place the patient in a stable side position, the recovery position.

- If the patient has a known paralyzed side, place that side down.

- Roll the patient gently into the recovery position, pulling the upper leg forward to prevent the patient from rolling onto his or her face.

- As with all unconscious patients, the recovery position maintains a critically important open airway.

to adequately manage his or her own airway. An open airway, as always, demands priority attention. Don't be surprised by a conscious patient who has lost the ability to speak or who has slurred speech or who complains of loss of memory. Breathing irregularities are not uncommon. Facial paralysis or facial drooping may be apparent, usually one-sided. *Hemiparesis* or *hemiplegia* (weakness or paralysis affecting one side of the body) is likely. Loss of reactivity in one pupil is not uncommon. Blurred or decreased vision in one eye may be a complaint. Incontinence may occur.

Supplemental Oxygen

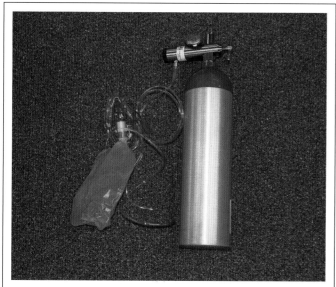

- A brain threatened by a stroke has the best chance when supplemental oxygen is delivered as soon as possible.

- Green is the color that indicates oxygen. The tank will be green or be banded in green.

- A full tank is stored at a pressure of two thousand pounds per square inch (PSI). A regulator is required to reduce the pressure and regulate the flow rate at which the oxygen is delivered.

- Stroke patients should receive the highest flow rate possible.

Note the Time!
- Note as precisely as possible the time of the onset of the stroke to assist physicians in determining the best course of medical action.

NEUROLOGICAL & DIABETIC

99

SEIZURE

Uncontrolled electrical activity in the brain causes seizures from mild to severe

A seizure is a discharge of uncontrolled electrical activity in the brain. There is an episode of involuntary behavior, which may or may not be associated with an altered mental state. Although more than twenty types of seizures have been identified, they can be classified as either partial or generalized.

For simplicity, *partial seizures* may be described as seizures affecting a localized part of the brain. Violent or jerking motions, if present, will be limited. The patient may stare blindly, wander aimlessly, or repeat a simple motor movement such as lip smacking. No emergency care is required other than careful monitoring of the patient to make sure that the seizure does not progress and/or that the patient is not endangered.

The Seizure 1

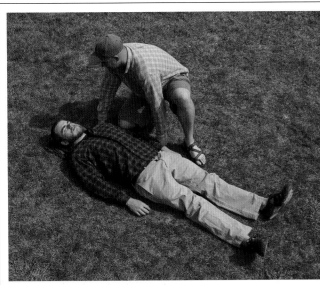

- During a seizure, the patient should *not* be restrained in any way, shape, or form.

- Place a protective pad underneath the patient's head to prevent damage to the head.

- Place protective padding over objects the patient may strike during the seizure, or place yourself between the patient and those objects. But be aware that the patient may strike violently.

- Patients may not breathe during a seizure, but they may be incontinent.

The Seizure 2

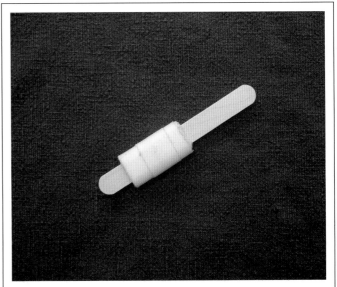

- Although bite sticks were once frequently used, you should place nothing in a patient's mouth during a seizure.

- If patients choose to place something in their own mouths prior to a seizure, that is entirely up to them.

- Patients may bite their tongues or the inside of their mouths during a seizure. That can be attended to later.

- Patients cannot swallow their tongues. It is a myth and anatomically impossible.

Generalized seizures, on the other hand, tend to be far more dramatic. Some patients describe an aura prior to their seizure, a "funny" feeling, a sick feeling, an odd taste or smell. An aura predicts a seizure. Tonic-clonic activity is the most dramatic presentation in a generalized seizure. The patient assumes a tonic (rigid) posture. The patient's head may turn to one side or be forced backward. Within less than a minute, typically, the patient enters the clonic (jerking) phase, rapidly thrashing around, striking the head and extremities on whatever happens to be in the way.

After the Seizure

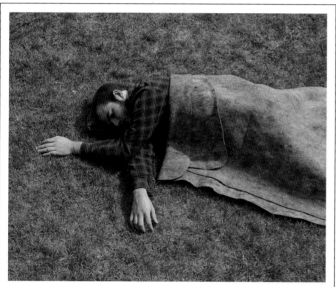

- The period following a seizure is called the "post-ictal phase."

- During this phase, the patient is typically exhausted and drowsy and may fall deeply asleep for forty-five minutes or more. The patient will later appreciate having had privacy in which to recover.

- Place this patient in the recovery position in order to safely maintain the airway.

- Assess the patient carefully for injuries—bruises, cuts, fractures—that could have occurred during the seizure.

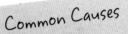

YELLOW LIGHT

Seizure disorders that cause mild seizures do not require a physician. First-time seizures, seizures without a known cause, and extended seizures should be evaluated by a physician.

Common Causes

- Seizure disorders
- High fever or heat stroke
- Brain injury
- Alcohol or drug withdrawal or overdose
- Diabetic hypoglycemia

NEUROLOGICAL & DIABETIC

DIABETES: HYPOGLYCEMIA

Hypoglycemia may strike suddenly and requires a quick and sure response

Diabetes is a complex disease involving sugar metabolism. The disease usually manifests as either too little sugar in the blood or too much. In some emergencies, first aid can save the life of a diabetic in need of help.

Hypoglycemia (low blood sugar) results from the treatment of diabetes, not the diabetes itself. Insulin-dependent diabetics must monitor their blood sugar (with a glucometer) and match injections of synthetic insulin to their food and activity level. Hypoglycemia can occur if the diabetic skips a meal but takes the usual insulin dose, takes more than the normal insulin dose, exercises strenuously and fails to eat, or vomits a meal after taking insulin. If a diabetic takes too much insulin and not enough

Insulin

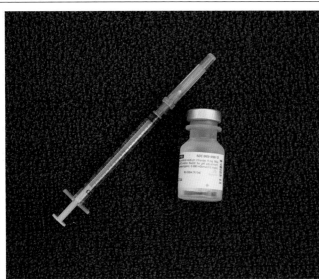

- In nondiabetic persons, insulin is made in the pancreas and released into the blood as needed to facilitate absorption of nutrients by cells.

- Diabetic persons make too little or no insulin.

- They have to inject insulin to match the food they eat and their level of exercise.

- Diabetics who do not match insulin to food and activity can suddenly find themselves life-threateningly low on blood sugar. The brain will not survive long without a constant supply of blood sugar.

Sugar

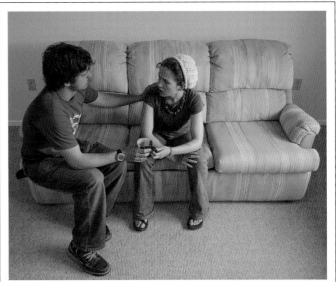

- Diabetics who need sugar are weak, disoriented, and irritable. They can become unresponsive and suffer a seizure.

- Their hearts speed up. Their breathing may remain normal, or it may become shallow. Their skin grows pale, cool, and sweaty.

- They need something sweet with simple sugars immediately! Sugar takes the least amount of time to become available in the blood.

- It is probably best if you can have the patient drink the sugar, such as adding sugar to a glass of orange juice.

food, the blood sugar level will be greatly depleted, insufficient to maintain normal brain function.

The onset of signs and symptoms is usually rapid and reflects the sensitivity of the brain to low blood sugar. Altered mental states—confusion, slurred speech, dizziness, nervousness, weakness, irritability—are typical early signs and symptoms. Other vital signs changes will include a rapid heart rate, normal or shallow respiratory rate, and pale, cool, and clammy skin. As the blood sugar drops, disorientation and unconsciousness can result.

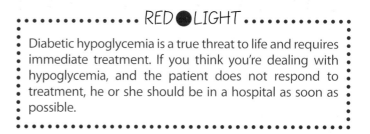

Eating a Meal

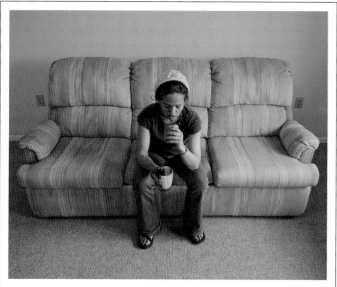

- It may take more time than you think it should, but eventually the patient will respond to sugar.

- Sometimes the change seems sudden: A patient may go from appearing "ill" to appearing "normal" in a matter of moments.

- Once appearing to have recovered, the patient needs to consume a meal or at least a hearty snack, encouraging the blood sugar level to stabilize.

- When the blood sugar level stabilizes, the patient will be ready to resume normal activities.

Unconsciousness and Sugar

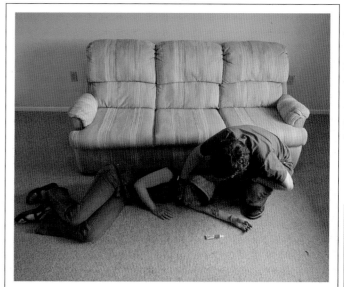

- The patient who has lapsed into an unresponsive state needs sugar even more critically than the conscious patient.

- This patient will be best attended to in a hospital. Call 911.

- In the meantime, you can give sugar by rolling the patient into a stable side position and rubbing sugar into the gums.

- You must repeatedly rub sugar or a sugar-rich substitute into the gums until the patient recovers or help arrives.

103

DIABETES: HYPERGLYCEMIA
Hyperglycemia tends to come on much more gradually than hypoglycemia

Diabetics who have defective or insufficient insulin can develop *hyperglycemia* (high blood sugar). Additionally, when diabetics become ill they are in danger of developing hyperglycemia as the body responds to the infection by increasing blood sugar levels. Without insulin, the kidneys work to excrete the abundance of sugar in the blood, along

with water and electrolytes, and the result is dehydration, electrolyte problems, and altered metabolism.

Hyperglycemia develops more slowly than hypoglycemia. The first symptoms are increased hunger, increased thirst, and an increased volume of urine output, and there may be nausea and vomiting. The patient's breath may have a fruity odor from

Glucometer

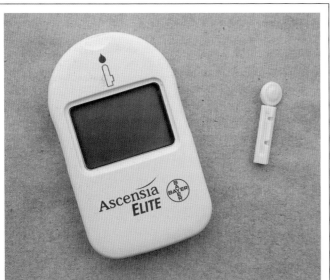

- Diabetics monitor their blood sugar level with a glucometer, a small, portable device that runs on batteries.

- They must prick their finger, draw a small drop of blood, and place the blood on a tiny plate on the glucometer.

- Normal blood sugar levels for diabetics and nondiabetics fall between 80 and 120 milligrams per deciliter (of blood).

- The number that appears on the tiny screen of the glucometer will indicate the amount of blood sugar in milligrams per deciliter.

Hydration

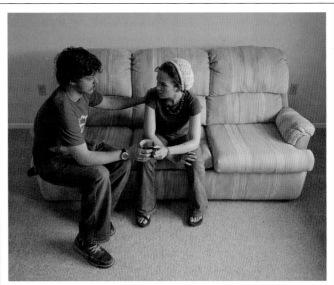

- The patient has too little insulin, and blood sugar, unable to be used, is collecting in the blood in ever-increasing amounts. The blood sugar level can reach into the hundreds!

- The breath will begin to smell sweet, sugary, like

- acetone, or somewhat alcoholic.

- The patient will be very thirsty and tired and will probably report an increased urine output.

- These persons need lots of fluids, especially water, to prevent dehydration.

the metabolism of fats as an energy source, the result of the body's demand for nutrition. There may be abdominal cramps and signs of dehydration that include flushed, dry skin.

The brain, which needs glucose almost as much as it needs oxygen, absorbs glucose freely from the blood. Because glucose is able to cross the brain/blood barrier without insulin, the onset of neurological changes is delayed, often taking days to appear. Loss of consciousness, therefore, is a late and very serious sign—although you can expect to see changes in mental function, such as attitude alterations, sooner.

Insulin

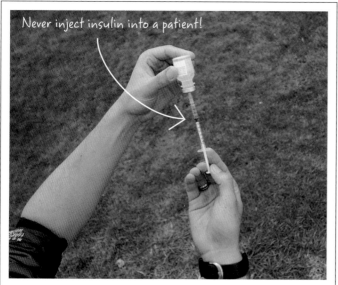

Never inject insulin into a patient!

- Although the hyperglycemic patient needs insulin, you must *never* give insulin to this patient!

- Insulin is not all the same. Some acts quickly, for instance, and some acts slowly. And the amount that must be given varies.

- If you can find the patient's insulin and syringes, and if the patient can check blood sugar and inject the proper amount of the proper insulin, that will be excellent.

- Otherwise make sure the patient is transported to a hospital.

The hyperglycemic patient has a complex problem, is dehydrated with an electrolyte imbalance, and needs the care of a physician. Never give insulin unless the patient is capable of administering the injection.

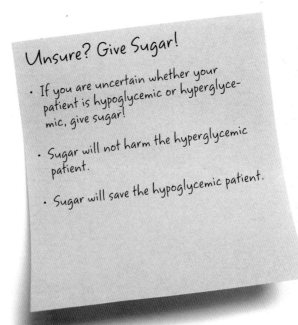

Unsure? Give Sugar!

- If you are uncertain whether your patient is hypoglycemic or hyperglycemic, give sugar!

- Sugar will not harm the hyperglycemic patient.

- Sugar will save the hypoglycemic patient.

NEUROLOGICAL & DIABETIC

105

PREVENTING DIABETIC EMERGENCIES

Unlike with many other diseases, preventive strategies can prevent most diabetic emergencies

You can take precautions to reduce the chance of a diabetic emergency to a minimum:

Encourage anyone with diabetes to stay in shape, a high level of physical fitness being an extremely important factor in the management of the disease.

Remind anyone with diabetes to stay well hydrated.

Diabetics should carry a readily available carbohydrate source, such as glucose tablets or gel.

If you are associated with a diabetic, learn how to use the glucometer. A reading of 80 to 120 is the normal range for blood sugar. Low readings may require sugar intake, and high readings suggest that insulin is needed.

Diabetic Kit

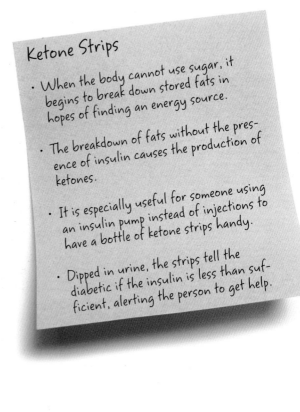

- Diabetics need to have a kit containing the items they need to manage their disease relatively close at all times.

- The kit should contain insulin, syringes, glucometer, spare batteries, lancets for drawing blood, and anything else needed to monitor and maintain blood sugar level.

- The kit may contain glucose tabs or gel or some other form of quick sugar.

- The kit may have a pocket for a cold pack. Insulin does not tolerate high temperatures.

Ketone Strips

- When the body cannot use sugar, it begins to break down stored fats in hopes of finding an energy source.

- The breakdown of fats without the presence of insulin causes the production of ketones.

- It is especially useful for someone using an insulin pump instead of injections to have a bottle of ketone strips handy.

- Dipped in urine, the strips tell the diabetic if the insulin is less than sufficient, alerting the person to get help.

Suggest that anyone with diabetes limit the use of concentrated sources of simple glucoses, such as candy. For snacks, suggest nutrient-dense foods such as nuts and dried fruits.

Remind anyone with diabetes not to skip meals.

On trips away from home, plan each day the night before, including wake-up time. Sleeping late can be adjusted for by merely pushing all meals back. Adjust for late dinners by switching the bedtime snack with the regular dinner time or by reducing the morning insulin dose and taking an evening injection of regular insulin just prior to the evening meal.

Food

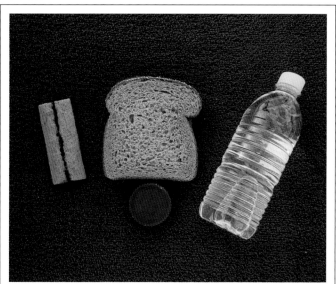

- To prevent diabetic emergencies, diabetics must monitor what and when they eat, balancing their food and exercise level with the amount of insulin they take.

- They can become unbalanced if they eat excessively and/or fail to exercise on a regular basis.

- They need to be especially careful to stay well hydrated at all times.

- They also need to be especially careful when fighting off an illness that can alter their normal use of food.

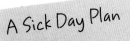
A Sick Day Plan

- Need to know how to adjust insulin for illness

- Need to know how to adjust food and fluid intake

- Need to monitor ketones in urine

- Need to take special precautions with diarrhea and/or vomiting

NEUROLOGICAL & DIABETIC

107

INGESTED POISONS

Swallowed poisons are the most common cause of poisoning emergencies

Children are the most common victims of serious poisoning. If you suspect poisoning, your best action is to call a poison control center for quick advice. Find the phone number, and keep it handy.

Limiting the absorption of the poison from the gastrointestinal tract of anyone who has ingested a poison is the prime goal of management. There are three practical methods of doing this: (1) diluting the poison with as much water as the patient will drink, (2) inducing vomiting, and (3) binding the toxin with activated charcoal.

If vomiting can be induced early, within one hour, it may be beneficial. Stimulation of the gag reflex typically works

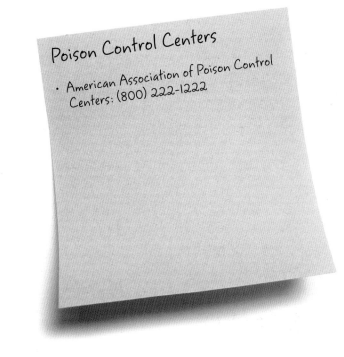

Poison Control Centers

• American Association of Poison Control Centers: (800) 222-1222

Vomiting

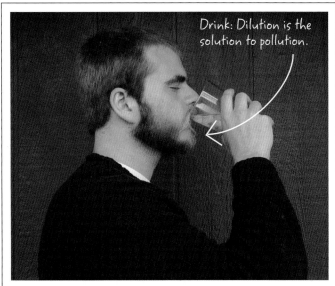

Drink: Dilution is the solution to pollution.

- If you can induce vomiting within approximately one hour of ingestion of a poison, it may be beneficial.

- Start by having the patient drink a glass of water.

- Do *not* induce vomiting if the patient is losing consciousness or if the patient has a seizure disorder or heart problems.

- Do not induce vomiting if the patient has swallowed corrosive acids or bases, both of which can increase damage as they come up, or if the patient has swallowed a petroleum product.

as well, or better, than anything else. Lean patients forward, ask them to stick their tongues out as far as possible, gently reach into their mouth with a finger, and tickle the back of their throat.

In the case of ingestion of corrosive chemicals or petroleum products, do not induce vomiting. Get the patient to drink a liter of water. Diluting the poison will reduce its effects.

Activated charcoal is postcombustion carbon residue treated to increase absorbency. With most poisons, even if your care will be short term, binding the toxins with charcoal may provide an even better treatment than inducing vomiting. Why? By the time you realize you have a poisoned patient, much of the toxin has already passed out of the stomach, and there are *no* contraindications for the use of activated charcoal. Charcoal may also be administered postvomiting.

If the patient goes unconscious, evacuation to a medical facility is probably what is going to save a life. Keep the patient on her or his side during the evacuation to maintain the airway.

Activated Charcoal

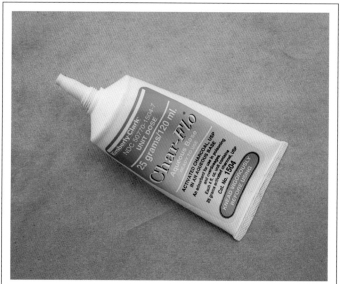

- Activated charcoal binds with many poisons, preventing the poison from being absorbed by the body. It can be found in almost any pharmacy without a prescription.

- The usual dose is 50–100 grams for adults and 20–50 grams for children.

- Although it is odorless and tasteless, swallowing the slurry of fine black powder may prove a chore.

- It can be added to flavored drinks (e.g., fruit drinks), but it should not be mixed with milk or milk products.

Ingested Poison Management

- Call the local poison control center.

- Encourage the patient to drink water to dilute the poison.

- Consider inducing vomiting.

- Consider activated charcoal.

INHALED POISONS

Poisons breathed in may cause serious breathing difficulties

Carbon monoxide (CO) poisonings account for approximately one-half the deaths by poison in the United States every year, making CO the leading cause of all fatal poisonings.

This invisible, odorless, tasteless, nonirritating gas is the result of incomplete combustion of any carbon-based fuel—gasoline, kerosene, natural gas, charcoal, and wood.

As the amount of carbon monoxide increases in the body to as little as 10 percent of the maximum potential, the patient develops a terrible headache, nausea, vomiting, and a loss of manual dexterity. At 30 percent the level of consciousness descends into irritability, impaired judgment, and confusion. It will be increasingly difficult for the patient to get a full breath, and he or she will grow drowsy. At 40–60 percent the patient lapses into a coma. Levels above 60 percent are usually fatal. The "cherry-red skin" often associated with the terminal stage of CO poisoning is, in truth, very rarely seen.

Carbon Monoxide

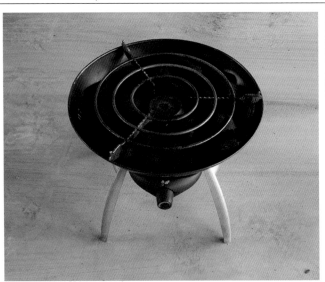

- Carbon monoxide is an odorless, tasteless, nonirritating, and invisible gas formed by the incomplete combustion of any carbon-based fuel.

- It is the leading cause of fatal poisonings in the United States and often associated with camping trips.

- CO binds aggressively to red blood cells, causing those blood cells to be unable to carry enough oxygen.

- If too many red blood cells are unable to carry oxygen, the patient suffers heart failure.

Fresh Air

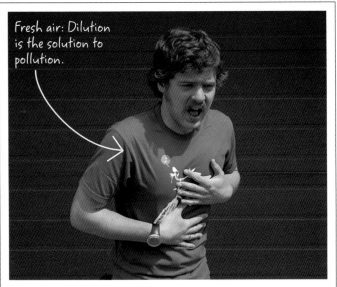

Fresh air: Dilution is the solution to pollution.

- The patient needs to be immediately removed from the source of any inhaled poison and moved into fresh air. Once breathing fresh air, most patients will eventually recover.

- Some poisons, especially carbon monoxide, do not cease their ill effects until hours after the patient is removed from the source.

- Any patient with an altered level of mental status after inhaling a poison or any patient who continues to be in respiratory distress requires rapid transport to a medical facility.

Death typically results from heart failure.

Move the patient to fresh air. After inhaling low concentrations of CO, the patient will probably recover completely in a few hours. If the concentrations have been high, the patient may die even if removed from the source of the gas. A high concentration of supplemental oxygen is the most important immediate treatment for severe poisoning by inhalation.

More First Aid

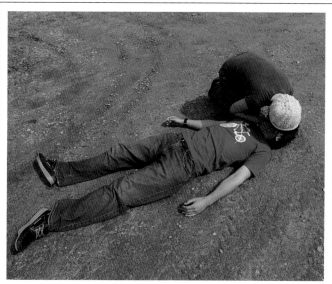

- Any patient who stops breathing after inhaling a poison needs rescue breathing immediately.

- Some patients suffering from an inhaled poison will complain of burning or watery eyes, sore throat, hoarseness or a cough— but remember that signs and symptoms do not always show right away.

- Any person suspected of inhaling a poison should be given supplemental oxygen as soon as it is available. The patient should be transported to a hospital for evaluation, even if he or she appears to have recovered.

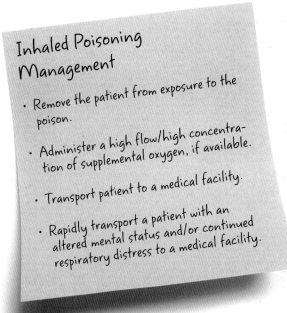

Inhaled Poisoning Management

- Remove the patient from exposure to the poison.

- Administer a high flow/high concentration of supplemental oxygen, if available.

- Transport patient to a medical facility.

- Rapidly transport a patient with an altered mental status and/or continued respiratory distress to a medical facility.

POISONING & ALLERGIES

ABSORBED POISONS

Poisons absorbed through the skin may contaminate the rescuer as well as the victim

Absorbed poisons are substances that cause tissue irritation or destruction after coming in contact with skin, eyes, or the lining of the nose, mouth, and throat.

Acids, alkalis, and hydrocarbons are the most destructive. Harmful chemicals are often found in fertilizers and pesticides. Some plant oils are considered absorbed poisons (see

"Contact Dermatitis"). Serious accidents are not usually seen outside of industrial and farming environments.

The first step in treatment is to get the patient out of contaminated clothing. Prevent the clothing, as much as possible, from touching bare skin. Liquid poisons should be dabbed off the skin with absorbent material. Dry poisons should be

Removal of Clothing

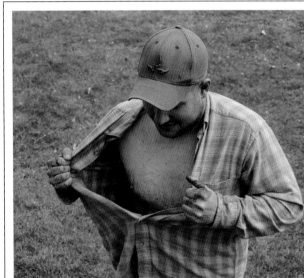

Flush

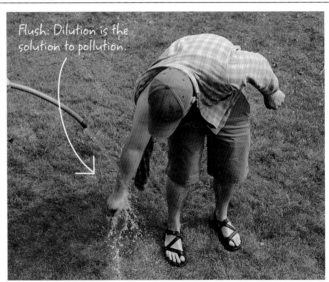

Flush: Dilution is the solution to pollution.

- Any patient who has contacted an absorbed poison should have all clothing that could have been contaminated removed immediately.

- As much as possible, prevent contact of the clothing with bare skin.

- To prevent contamination to yourself, allow the patient to remove clothing without your assistance, if possible.

- All poison visible on skin should be immediately brushed off without additional contact with skin. You can use uncontaminated clothing as a brush.

- Damage from some absorbed poisons can be severe.

- All skin that could have contacted the poison should be immediately flushed with running water for at least ten minutes.

- If the poison entered the

eyes, the eyes should be flushed with running water: ten minutes for an acid and twenty minutes for an alkali.

- A few poisons, such as phosphorus and elemental sodium, are activated by water. These can be only brushed off. Do *not* flush.

112

brushed off. Most victims of absorbed poisons should now be flushed with clean water (which is why you see emergency showers at many industrial sites). Flushing should be continuous for approximately ten minutes, or twenty minutes if the poison was an alkali. Flushing should include eyes, nose, and mouth if those are involved.

Be aware that some poisons, such as phosphorus, are activated by water and should not be flushed off.

All patients contaminated with destructive poisons should then be transported to a hospital.

Wash

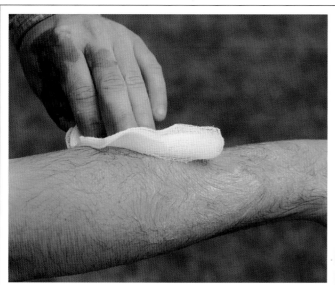

- All patients who have contacted an absorbed poison should be transported to a hospital as soon as possible after flushing.

- If possible, it is beneficial to continue flushing of the affected area during transport.

- If transport is delayed, the patient should wash contaminated skin with soap and water after flushing. Repeat the wash with soap and water at least once.

- If transport is delayed, contact the local poison control center for further advice.

Absorbed Poisoning Management

- As a first-aid provider, avoid contact with the poison.

- Remove contaminated clothing.

- Flush with water for at least ten minutes.

- If transport is delayed, wash with soap and water.

113

POISONING & ALLERGIES

MILD ALLERGIES

The allergens that cause allergies may be ingested, inhaled, absorbed, or injected

An *allergic reaction* results from an acquired hypersensitivity to a substance that causes no reaction in the great majority of people. The allergy-causing substance is called an "allergen." Mild allergies are very common and, as the name implies, not serious. Allergic reactions are caused by an excessive release of histamines and other substances from the body's immune system in response to the presence of allergens. A relatively small release of histamine causes mild to moderate signs and symptoms.

Most common are patients who suffer seasonal "hay fevers." The reaction begins as an itch in the nose—gradually or abruptly—just after the onset of pollen season. It spreads,

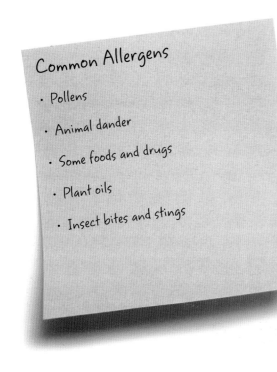

Common Allergens

- Pollens
- Animal dander
- Some foods and drugs
- Plant oils
- Insect bites and stings

Contact

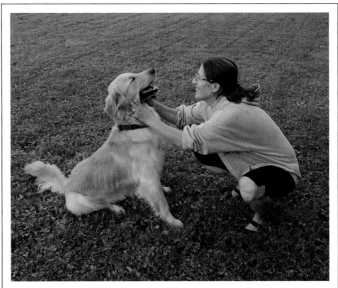

- As with known poisons, allergens are contacted via ingestion, inhalation, absorption, or injection.

- Unlike known poisons, allergens do not cause a reaction in a majority of people. In sensitive people, allergens cause a mild to moderate overreaction in their immune system. The primary overreaction is an overproduction of histamines.

- The overreaction may produce watery and itchy eyes and/or nose, coughing, sneezing, and flushed and itchy skin—but no pronounced respiratory difficulty.

usually, to the eyes and the roof of the mouth and the back of the throat. Eyes begin to water, and the patient begins to sneeze. Hacking cough, headache, rash, loss of appetite, lack of sleep, depression, and irritability may be seen or described by the patient. The patient may complain of a feeling of tightness in the chest, and you may hear a whistling sound, a wheeze, when the patient takes a breath.

About 95 percent of all allergy medications contain the same ingredients, and they can be divided into two categories: antihistamines and decongestants.

Antihistamines

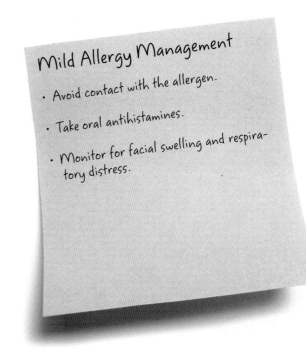
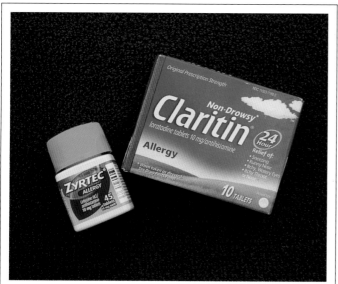

- Histamines are a critically important part of your immune system. They support the body's response to the invasion of foreign substances, such as bacteria.

- Too many histamines, however, are the primary cause of the signs and symptoms of an allergy.

- Over-the-counter antihistamines counteract the effects of an overproduction of histamines.

- As with all medications, you should read and carefully follow the directions on the labels unless otherwise directed by your physician.

Mild Allergy Management

- Avoid contact with the allergen.

- Take oral antihistamines.

- Monitor for facial swelling and respiratory distress.

POISONING & ALLERGIES

CONTACT DERMATITIS
Poison ivy, oak, and sumac cause most allergic reactions of the skin

The most common contact dermatitis results from urushiol, the oil in poison ivy, oak, and sumac. About 50 percent of all adults in the United States are very sensitive. Another 35 percent will have a reaction to higher concentrations of urushiol. The rest do not react, even to extremely high concentrations.

When urushiol soaks into sensitive human skin, an allergic reaction takes place. Most people first develop redness where they contacted the oil. The redness often appears in streaks where the plant brushed the skin. There may be swelling. Blisters, sometimes large, sometimes small, erupt later and discharge the fluid that fills them. The discharge will eventually form a crust. The entire area itches with indescribable ferocity.

Of prime importance is washing as soon as possible after contact has occurred. Cold water deactivates urushiol. If you

The Plants

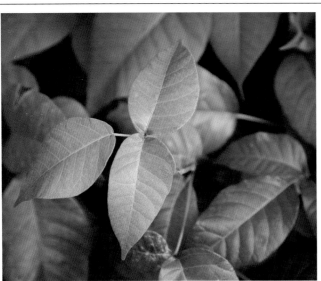

- Poison ivy is a plant found in much of the United States, but its appearance varies greatly depending on its location.

- There are two varieties of poison oak: eastern and western. The western plants cause more reactions in humans because they are far more ubiquitous.

- Poison sumac is a tree growing in the eastern United States in wet or flooded ground, most often in swamps.

- You need to be able to identify these plants in your area.

Washing

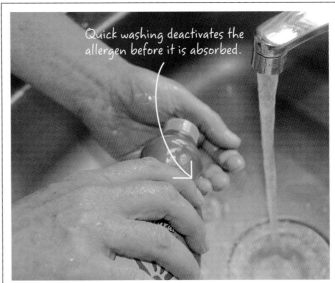

Quick washing deactivates the allergen before it is absorbed.

- Immediate washing with cold water—within three minutes after contact—will deactivate the highly irritating oil of these plants.

- After three minutes, you should wash—as soon as possible—with soap and cool to cold water.

- Avoid hard soaps. Most soft soaps will work, and liquid dish and laundry soaps have proven effective.

- Repeat the washing with soap and cool to cold water five or six times with adequate rinsing between the washings.

116

have plenty of cold water available, especially within the first three minutes of contact, soap is not required. Avoid hot water, which may spread the oil around more than off and/or open the pores so that the oil soaks in faster.

Washing with soap and water is recommended after the three-minute period ends. As to what kind of soap, the experts vary in exact recommendations, but detergents—such as dish and laundry—seem to work as well as anything. Of greater importance than what kind of soap is how you use it: Use five or six repeated rubbings, not aggressive scrubbings, with sufficient rinses between.

Organic solvents such as alcohol and gasoline work even better than water or soap and water. The preferred method is to dab repeatedly with several pieces of solvent-soaked cotton to pick up urushiol from the skin before giving the skin a good rub with fresh solvent-soaked cotton.

The Reaction

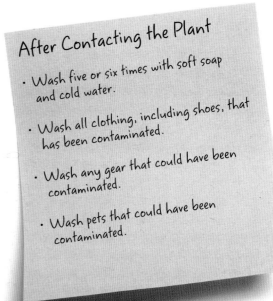

- There is no cure for the allergic reaction to the oil in these plants, but you will want to treat the symptoms, primarily the itching.

- Many people get some relief from the itching by applying a thin layer of 1 percent hydrocortisone cream or calamine lotion, both available over the counter.

- Oral antihistamines available over the counter may also help reduce the itching.

- It takes around ten days for the allergic reaction to run its course.

After Contacting the Plant

- Wash five or six times with soft soap and cold water.

- Wash all clothing, including shoes, that has been contaminated.

- Wash any gear that could have been contaminated.

- Wash pets that could have been contaminated.

117

SEVERE ALLERGIES

Anaphylaxis, a severe allergic reaction, can cause death in minutes

Anaphylaxis is a true, life-threatening emergency. It often begins like a general allergic reaction but rapidly results in respiratory and/or circulatory collapse. The onset of the signs and symptoms of anaphylaxis typically occurs within minutes of a bite or sting and within thirty to sixty minutes of ingestion of an allergen.

The signs and symptoms of anaphylaxis usually involve flushing, itching, burning, and swelling of the skin, especially of the face. The tongue may swell. There is extreme difficulty breathing. You may see signs and symptoms of shock (see "Shock").

If you suspect that a person susceptible to anaphylaxis has been exposed to a known allergen, give an oral antihistamine as soon as possible, a treatment that might forestall the anaphylactic reaction.

The ability to reverse fatal anaphylaxis requires the admin-

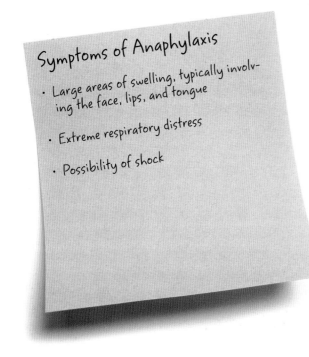

Symptoms of Anaphylaxis

- Large areas of swelling, typically involving the face, lips, and tongue

- Extreme respiratory distress

- Possibility of shock

Epinephrine

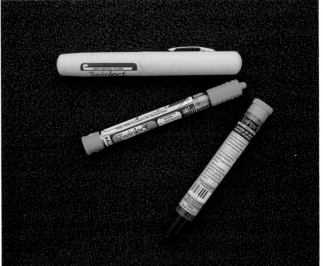

- Only epinephrine administered by way of an injection reverses the life threat of anaphylaxis.

- Epinephrine is available only with a prescription, and it should be acquired and carried by all individuals with a known susceptibility to anaphylaxis.

- An EpiPen is a spring-loaded auto-injector that delivers one dose of epinephrine.

- A Twinject can deliver two doses of epinephrine, the first a spring-loaded auto-injection, and the second requiring manual injection of the drug.

istration of injectable epinephrine. Epinephrine, once injected, works to reverse the respiratory distress and shock. This prescription-only product is available in kit form, and two products are available. One is the EpiPen, a spring-loaded auto-injector that is pressed into the outer thigh. Injecting through clothing works. The other is the Twinject, with two injections, the first an auto-injected dose, and the second requiring manual injection. Many persons with a history of severe allergic reactions will have one of these kits prescribed for their use by their physician.

Use of Auto-Injectors

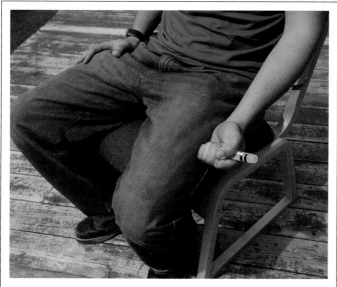

- Auto-injectors have a safety cap that must be removed prior to use.

- When pressed into the outer thigh, the spring-loaded dose of epinephrine is automatically delivered. It will go through clothing.

- The dose is delivered in seconds, but you should hold the auto-injector in place for ten seconds to be sure.

- An auto-injector should never be held with your thumb over the end. If you accidentally hold it backward, it will inject your thumb.

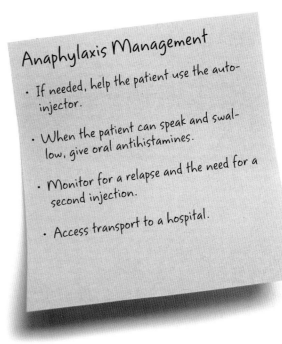

Anaphylaxis Management

- If needed, help the patient use the auto-injector.

- When the patient can speak and swallow, give oral antihistamines.

- Monitor for a relapse and the need for a second injection.

- Access transport to a hospital.

POISONING & ALLERGIES

STOMACHACHE

This complaint may be the most common symptom in humans

"Stomachache" is a word that means many things, depending on who is complaining about what. Medically speaking, there are approximately three hundred known causes of stomachache, ranging from indigestion to stomach cancer. The stomach, in fact, may not even be involved. Stomachache is often, for instance, distress in the intestines. Fortunately, most stomachaches are not serious.

Many stomachaches that require treatment present sim-ilarly. There is often intermittent cramping, usually worse in the lower abdomen. The pain is typically diffuse, not concentrated at one point. The stomach may "grumble." There may be nausea, vomiting, and/or diarrhea, covered later in this section. There may be a low fever.

The patient needs to be kept hydrated. Clear fluids are essential in helping the body overcome the germs. A bland diet is recommended, such as bananas, rice, applesauce, and

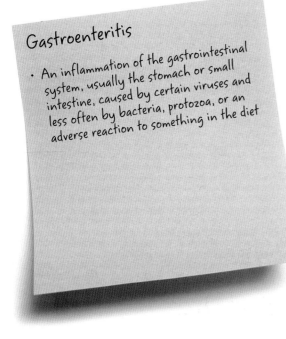

Gastroenteritis

- An inflammation of the gastrointestinal system, usually the stomach or small intestine, caused by certain viruses and less often by bacteria, protozoa, or an adverse reaction to something in the diet

Bland Diet

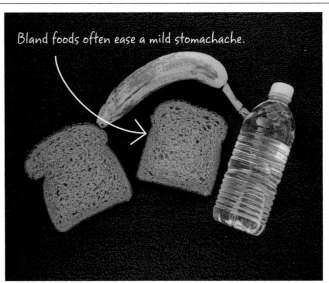

Bland foods often ease a mild stomachache.

- A bland diet is recommended for most people with a stomachache.

- The purpose of a bland diet is to decrease activity in the gastrointestinal system and to avoid irritation of the gastrointestinal tract.

- The foods of a bland diet are easy to digest, tender, and only mildly seasoned. Avoid fried foods, highly seasoned foods, and alcohol.

- Acceptable foods include milk, cottage cheese, fruits (especially bananas and avocados), squash, beans, peas, mushrooms, potatoes, and most breads.

toast. Avoid alcohol, dairy products, rich desserts, and spicy foods. Over-the-counter antidiarrheal and antiemetic (anti-vomiting) medications may be given, following the directions on the labels.

If the stomach is merely "upset," an antacid may be all the patient requires.

For information on deciding if a stomachache is serious, see "Severe Abdominal Illnesses."

······················ RED ● LIGHT ·····················

Persistent or worsening pain over twenty-four hours, the inability to tolerate fluids, blood in the stool, and/or a fever of 102°F or higher are signs that the patient needs to see a doctor.

Medications

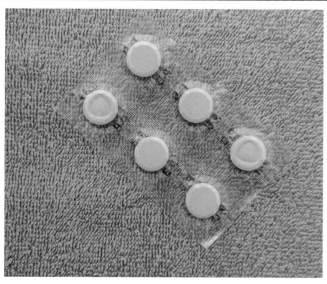

- Numerous medications are available over the counter and should be chosen depending on your symptoms. Read the labels carefully, and/or ask your pharmacist for advice.

- Chewable tablets that absorb stomach acid are often useful, as are medica-tions for diarrhea and nausea and medications that help relieve the buildup of pressure from gas.

- If you are taking a medication prescribed by your doctor, do not stop taking it while you manage your stomachache.

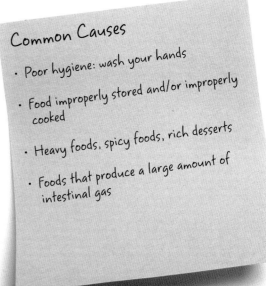

Common Causes

- Poor hygiene: wash your hands

- Food improperly stored and/or improperly cooked

- Heavy foods, spicy foods, rich desserts

- Foods that produce a large amount of intestinal gas

DIARRHEA

It's always unpleasant, but it can be serious if it is persistent

The world is home to a multitude of diarrhea-causing life forms. They will produce, generally speaking, one of two kinds of diarrhea: (1) *noninvasive diarrhea*, with microbial colonies on upper small intestine walls, leading to abdominal cramping, nausea, vomiting, and massive amounts of water, filled with salt and potassium, rushing out of the bowels, and (2) *invasive diarrhea*, sometimes called "dysentery," with bacteria attacking the lower small intestine and colon, causing

inflammation, bloody bowel movements, fever, abdominal cramping, and painful release of loose stools.

Whatever the cause, dehydration is the immediate problem with diarrhea. Mild diarrhea can be treated with water, diluted clear fruit juices, or sports drinks. Persistent diarrhea requires more aggressive replacement of electrolytes lost in the stool. Oral rehydration solutions, available over the counter, are best for treating serious diarrhea. You can get by,

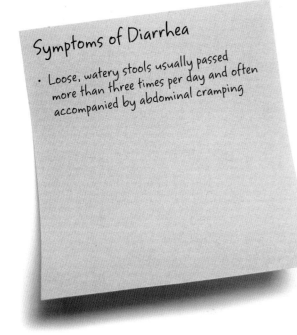

Symptoms of Diarrhea

· Loose, watery stools usually passed more than three times per day and often accompanied by abdominal cramping

Treatment 1

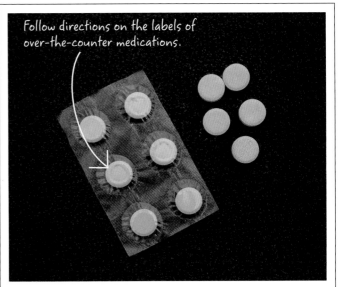

Follow directions on the labels of over-the-counter medications.

- Medications are available over the counter, and they often aid in the management of diarrhea.

- Medications are *not* recommended for treatment of diarrhea caused by bacteria or parasites unless prescribed by a doctor.

- Avoid foods that are greasy, high in fiber, and high in sugar. Avoid caffeine and milk products. These all may aggravate diarrhea.

- After improvement, limit your diet to bland foods such as bananas, plain rice, boiled potatoes, and toast.

usually, adding one teaspoon of salt and eight teaspoons of sugar to a liter of water. The patient should drink about one-fourth of this solution every hour, along with all the water he or she will tolerate. Rice, grains, bananas, and potatoes are okay to eat. Fats, dairy products, caffeine, and alcohol should be avoided.

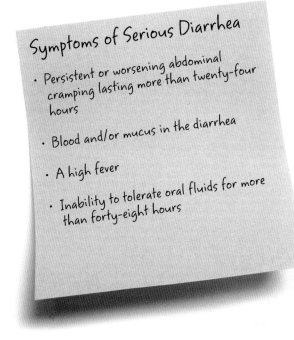

············· RED ● LIGHT ·············

Depending on the severity, diarrhea that lasts between twenty-four and seventy-two hours should be treated by a physician. The risk of severe dehydration may become a potential threat to life.

Treatment 2

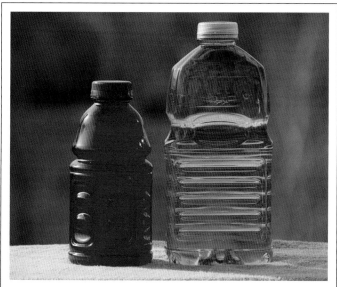

- It is critical to avoid dehydration when a person, especially a child or older adult, has diarrhea.

- When too much fluid and too many electrolytes are lost, the body cannot function properly.

- Water is essential in preventing diarrhea, but it does not contain electrolytes.

- Broth and soups that contain sodium, as well as clear fruit juices, may be consumed. Sports drinks also contain electrolytes. Over-the-counter rehydration solutions are valuable, especially with children.

Symptoms of Serious Diarrhea

- Persistent or worsening abdominal cramping lasting more than twenty-four hours

- Blood and/or mucus in the diarrhea

- A high fever

- Inability to tolerate oral fluids for more than forty-eight hours

123

CONSTIPATION

The inability to have a bowel movement is uncomfortable if mild and debilitating if persistent

Constipation is infrequent and/or difficult movement of the bowels, usually created by either an internal fluid level too low to lubricate the lower gastrointestinal tract and/or a fiber level too low to keep things rolling along. And constipation can be encouraged by poor exercise habits.

Treatment should start with forcing fluids, water being,

overall, the best lubricant. Encourage the patient to eat lots of whole grains, fruits (dried is okay), and vegetables. Peanut butter, cheese, and high-fat foods should be avoided. If a person is prone to the problem, add a stool softener—preferably a suppository—to your first-aid kit.

Stimulating the gastrocolic reflex will sometimes work to

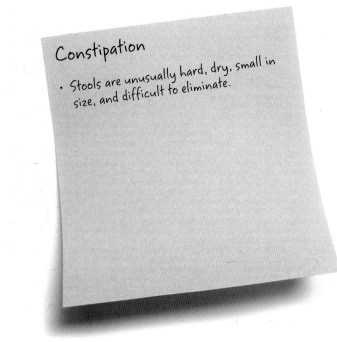

Constipation

• Stools are unusually hard, dry, small in size, and difficult to eliminate.

Fiber

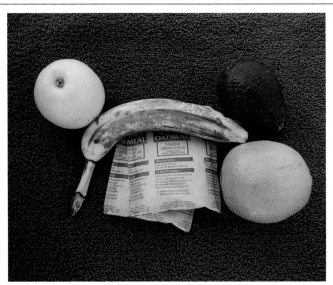

• Fiber is the parts of fruits, vegetables, and grains that the body cannot digest.

• People consuming diets high in fiber are far less likely to develop constipation.

• People consuming low-fiber diets, diets high in fats

such as cheese, eggs, and meat, are far more likely to develop constipation.

• Foods that are quick to make or buy, such as prepared foods, refined and processed foods, and fast foods, are usually low in fiber.

relieve constipation. Have the patient drink water, at least a half a liter, followed by a cup of hot coffee or tea.

Someone who hasn't had a bowel movement in three days typically feels uncomfortable. A patient without a movement in five days could be developing serious problems from the toxins building up in the intestinal tract. The problem could be a fecal impaction, requiring a visit to a hospital. In extreme emergencies, it might be necessary to go in with a lubricated, gloved index finger to break up the impaction, piece by piece, and pull it out. Disgusting as it may sound, it might prove life-saving.

ZOOM

Prevention of constipation in most people includes drinking plenty of fluids daily, especially water, and eating a healthy diet, one rich in fiber: fresh vegetables and fruit and whole grains.

Liquids

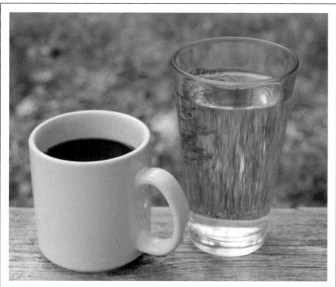

- Liquids add bulk to stools and fluid to the colon, making bowel movements softer and easier to pass.

- Liquids do sometimes but not always help relieve constipation, but they always help prevent constipation.

- Liquids high in caffeine

and alcoholic beverages do not help hydrate the body. Drinking plenty of water may counteract the dehydrating effect of caffeine and alcohol.

- A bowel movement may be encouraged by drinking a large glass of water followed by a cup of hot tea.

Medications

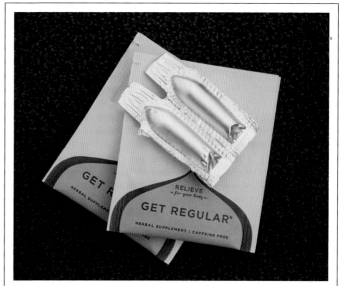

- Most people experiencing mild constipation do not need a laxative. Laxatives should not be taken indiscriminately.

- If lifestyle changes (more exercise) and diet changes (more fiber and liquids) do not relieve constipation, a doctor may recommend

over-the-counter laxatives.

- Laxatives do not all work the same way, and a doctor can tell you which laxative will probably be best for you.

- Under a doctor's care, laxatives can help retrain a sluggish bowel.

NAUSEA & VOMITING

Nausea is an unpleasant feeling, but vomiting can lead to serious dehydration

Nausea and vomiting, a pair of ugly cousins, can have many causes. Infections somewhere in the gastrointestinal tract, lumped under the name "gastroenteritis," typically viral, are a prevalent source. Then there's bad food, motion sickness, and altitude illness (see "Acute Mountain Sickness"). Usually the illness is just the body's way of dealing with something that is

upsetting the normal balance—and it is usually not serious.

But protracted vomiting can lead to dehydration and electrolyte imbalances. You can give the patient an antiemetic (antivomiting) medication, one available over the counter. Oral drugs are popular, but suppositories might be necessary because the patient might vomit up an oral drug before it has a chance to

The Queasy Feeling

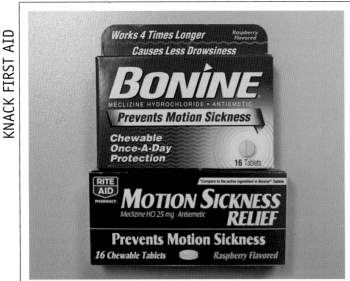

- Nausea, the urge to vomit, and vomiting, the forceful expulsion of the contents of the stomach, are usually the stomach's way of dealing with undesirable contents.

- They are one of the body's ways of protecting you from potential dangers and seldom require urgent

medical attention.

- Over-the-counter bismuth stomach remedies or another antivomiting drug may be useful. Bismuth remedies contain an aspirin-like substance and should not be taken by children unless they are under a doctor's care.

Motion Sickness

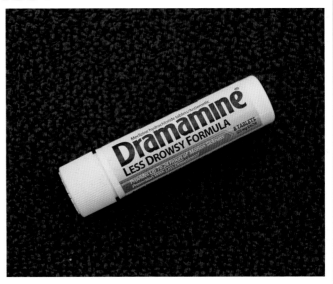

- Motion causes nausea and vomiting in large numbers of people.

- Sufferers sometimes find relief by lying down or choosing a location that reduces motion, such as in the middle of a boat or between the wings of a large airplane. Focusing on

a distant, nonmoving point can also be helpful.

- Over-the-counter antihistamines such as Dramamine prevent motion sickness in many people.

- Doctors may prescribe scopolamine patches for special cases.

126

work. Once the vomiting has stopped, ask the patient to keep drinking plenty of clear liquids: water and clear fruit juices.

People who suffer nausea regularly might find relief only from a prescription-strength drug, requiring a visit to a doctor. If any drug is taken for nausea resulting from motion, the drug must be taken prior to exposure to motion to be effective.

Vomitus should be inspected for the presence of blood. It will appear either as reddish vomit or, if partially digested, as dark "coffee grounds." The presence of blood is a signal to find a physician.

· · · · · · · · · · · · · RED ● LIGHT · · · · · · · · · · · · · ·

Vomiting may become a serious threat via dehydration if it persists for more than twenty-four hours. The more often vomiting occurs, the more serious the threat. Consult a physician about profound vomiting.

Hydration

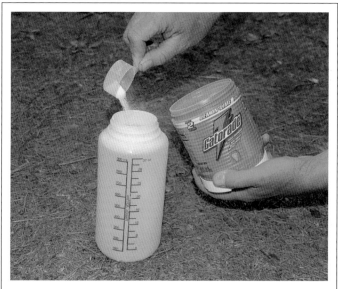

- Dehydration is the primary and potentially most serious complication of vomiting.

- How fast an individual dehydrates depends on the person's size and the frequency of vomiting.

- Water, clear fruit juices, sports drinks, or ginger ale should be consumed regularly. Electrolyte solutions are also helpful.

- Drink only small amounts. Large amounts stretch the stomach, often making vomiting worse. Do not eat solid foods until there has been no vomiting for at least six hours.

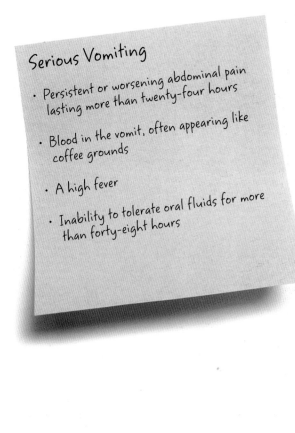

Serious Vomiting

- Persistent or worsening abdominal pain lasting more than twenty-four hours

- Blood in the vomit, often appearing like coffee grounds

- A high fever

- Inability to tolerate oral fluids for more than forty-eight hours

SEVERE ABDOMINAL ILLNESSES
You may not know the cause, but you need to know if it's serious

Even skilled physicians who specialize in abdominal problems may be unsure of the cause of the distress in the patient. There is much that can go wrong in the abdominal area of the body. What you need to assess is this: Is the pain serious, requiring a hospital?

Beware of abdominal pain associated with the signs and symptoms of shock (see "Shock").

Beware of abdominal pain that persists for longer than a period of twelve to twenty-four hours.

Beware if the pain localizes, concentrates in a specific area of the abdomen, and especially if the pain involves guarding (the patient voluntarily or involuntarily protects the area), tenderness, abdominal rigidity, and/or distention.

Beware if blood appears in the vomit, feces, or urine. In vomit blood may look like coffee grounds, in the stool it may look black like tar, in the urine it may be a reddish color.

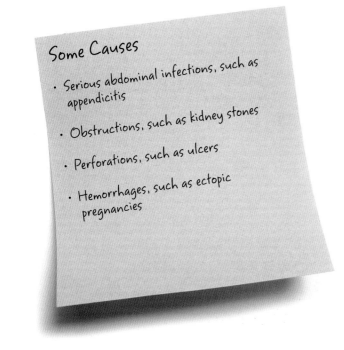

Some Causes

- Serious abdominal infections, such as appendicitis

- Obstructions, such as kidney stones

- Perforations, such as ulcers

- Hemorrhages, such as ectopic pregnancies

Position of Comfort

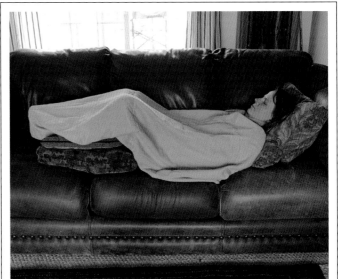

- Patients with severe abdominal pain need to be kept in a position that provides the most comfort. They should be kept covered to prevent loss of body heat.

- Straightening the legs often increases the abdominal pain, another sign that the pain could be serious.

- Patients may be kept in a side position with their legs flexed.

- They may be kept lying down with thick padding, such as pillows, beneath the knees.

Beware if the pain is associated with nausea, vomiting, and/or diarrhea that persists for longer than a period of twenty-four to seventy-two hours, especially if the patient is unable to stay well hydrated.

Beware if the pain is associated with a fever above 102°F.

Beware if the pain is associated with the signs and symptoms of pregnancy.

And beware if the patient complains of increased pain when a foot strikes the ground during walking.

ZOOM

If you decide that the patient's abdominal condition is serious, transport should be gentle, with the patient kept warm and in a position of greatest comfort. The patient should ingest nothing.

Hydration

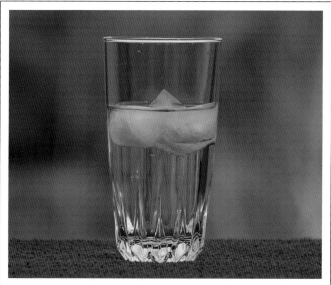

- In almost all cases, patients with severe abdominal pain should not be given anything to swallow, including water.

- However, in situations where transportation will be delayed for an extended period of time, dehydration must be avoided.

- If the patient is alert, small sips of cold water are usually tolerated and are unlikely to be harmful.

- If the patient complains of nausea, reduce the amount and/or the temperature of the water being given.

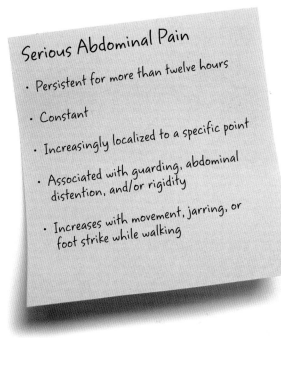

Serious Abdominal Pain

- Persistent for more than twelve hours

- Constant

- Increasingly localized to a specific point

- Associated with guarding, abdominal distention, and/or rigidity

- Increases with movement, jarring, or foot strike while walking

PREVENTING ABDOMINAL PROBLEMS
Most mild to moderate abdominal illnesses can be prevented

The mild to moderate abdominal problems that plague people can be avoided, to a large degree, with good hygiene.

Human hands are the primary vectors for germs that make people sick. Hand washing should be regular and adequate, especially after bowel movements and prior to food preparation. Hands should be scrubbed with soap and warm water for approximately thirty seconds, rinsed thoroughly, and dried thoroughly.

When using any water from a natural source, it needs to be disinfected. Bringing water to the boiling point will adequately disinfect it. Devices that use ultraviolet light work well to disinfect water. Water filters work to varying degrees—some filter a few harmful germs, some filter out most germs. Reading the label carefully before purchasing is critical. Chemicals that disinfect water will kill most harmful germs, with *Cryptosporidium* being a notable exception. Once again,

Hand Washing

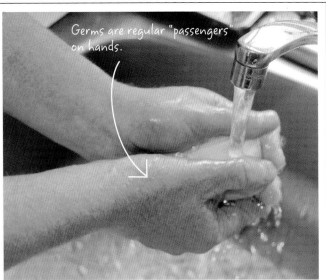

Germs are regular "passengers" on hands.

- Germs carried on hands are probably the primary source of abdominal discomfort.

- Hands should be washed after a person goes to the bathroom and before a person prepares food or provides first aid.

- Warm water works best.

- Use a soap that lathers up, then scrub, rinse, and dry your hands. Drying removes germs left on hands after washing.

- Keep your fingernails trimmed short, and clean under them regularly to further prevent the spread of disease.

Hand Sanitizers

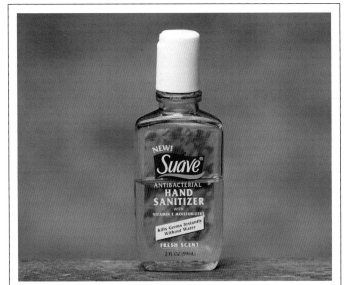

- In situations where water and soap are in short supply, you can keep your hands relatively free of germs with hand sanitizers.

- Sanitizers should be rubbed into the skin of your hands, and your hands should *not* be dried afterward.

- Sanitizers that contain moisturizers prevent your skin from drying out, a potential problem with extended use.

- Even when using sanitizers, try to use water and soap to wash your hands at least once a day.

reading the labels on products is important. Poorer filters can be used in concert with chemicals to guarantee safe water.

Keep perishable foods stored in the refrigerator. Store them as soon as possible after purchasing. Do not eat leftovers unless they have been refrigerated after serving.

Water Disinfection

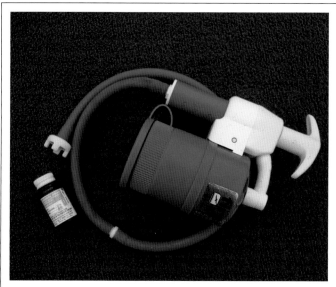

- In some situations, you may be required to disinfect drinking water in order to prevent waterborne illnesses.

- When a heat source is available, water brought to the point of a rolling boil is safe to drink.

- Some water filters remove all germs except viruses. Chemical disinfectants, such as iodine, kill all bacteria and viruses. With both methods, be sure to read the directions carefully.

- Devices that use ultraviolet light to disinfect water kill all germs.

Food

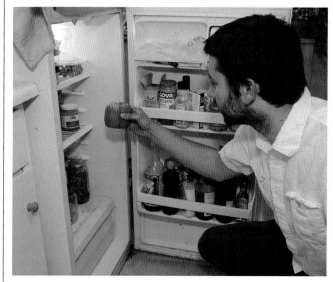

- Improperly stored and improperly cooked foods are often sources of abdominal illness.

- Perishable foods that require refrigeration should be refrigerated as soon as possible after purchasing.

- Leftovers should not be eaten unless stored at less than 45°F. In most cases, it is best to reheat leftovers before consumption.

- Follow the directions concerning cooking times on packaged foods. Note and take heed of the expiration dates on packaged foods.

MILD HYPOTHERMIA

Treat a small drop in body core temperature before it becomes big

Without doing anything active, the human body still makes heat via basal metabolism, the energy required to sustain life at complete rest. Add activity, anything powered by voluntary muscles, and the rate of internal heat production goes up. How much it goes up depends on the level of fitness of the individual and how hard that person is exercising.

Internal heat constantly flows from each person into the environment via radiation, evaporation, conduction, and convection. When humans lose body heat faster than they make heat, their body core temperature—normally about 98.6°F—may begin to drop, leading to a condition called "hypothermia." Mild hypothermia causes an individual to be, essentially, cold and unhappy. Greater losses of internal heat can cause death.

Medically speaking, hypothermia starts when a core temperature has dropped 3–4°F. At that point, the patient may

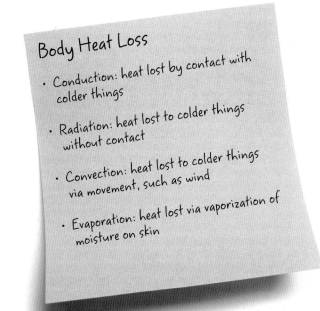

Body Heat Loss

- Conduction: heat lost by contact with colder things

- Radiation: heat lost to colder things without contact

- Convection: heat lost to colder things via movement, such as wind

- Evaporation: heat lost via vaporization of moisture on skin

Treatment 1

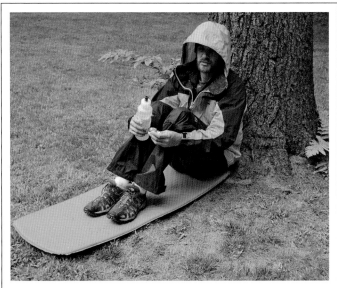

- The essential goal in the treatment of mild hypothermia is to change the patient's environment from wet and cold to dry and warm.

- Additional layers of clothing can be added over clothing that is not too wet.

- A layer that blocks wind prevents further heat loss via convection. The patient needs to be insulated from the ground.

- Assume hypothermic patients are at least somewhat dehydrated, so give them water to drink. A warm, sweet drink is best.

132

be described as suffering "a case of the umbles": stumbling during walking, then fumbling with tasks that require fine motor skills (such as zipping up a zipper), then grumbling (and becoming less and less sociable), and then mumbling while speaking.

Shivering, an involuntary form of exercise, is common. When shivering becomes violent and uncontrollable, the core temperature has usually dropped about 8–10 F, and the risk to the patient has risen.

Treatment 2

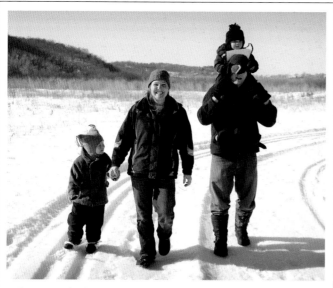

- Patients who have started to shiver uncontrollably are best treated by rest after they are protected from the environment.

- They also need fuel for their internal fires, something sweet that is turned into energy soon after being eaten.

- Patients, however, who are cold and not violently shivering can continue to exercise after eating, drinking, and putting on dry clothes.

- The patient who feels and acts normal once again has recovered from mild hypothermia.

Symptoms of Mild Hypothermia

- Fumbling: impaired ability to do complex tasks

- Stumbling: altered gait

- Mumbling: slurred speech

- Grumbling: sluggish thinking

- Shivering, but not uncontrollably

133

SEVERE HYPOTHERMIA

Mismanagement of a seriously cold person can make the problem more serious

When someone has depleted his or her stored energy and/or cooled off internally to the point where shivering stops, that person has developed severe hypothermia. You will see increasing muscular rigidity and stupor progressing to unconsciousness. The patient's heart rate will slow and weaken, eventually becoming undetectable. The respiratory rate will slow down and grow so shallow that it, too, is undetectable. Skin will turn deeply cold to the touch. Yet, that person is still alive.

Of the utmost importance is extra-gentle handling of the patient—even if the patient appears dead. Rough handling is likely to cause a weak, cold, fragile heart to stop.

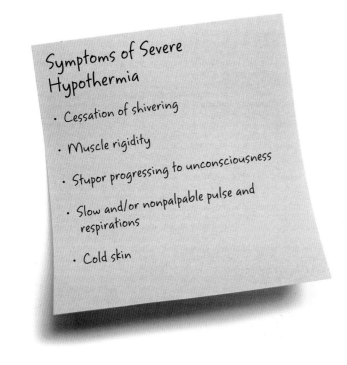

Symptoms of Severe Hypothermia

- Cessation of shivering
- Muscle rigidity
- Stupor progressing to unconsciousness
- Slow and/or nonpalpable pulse and respirations
- Cold skin

Hypothermia Wrap

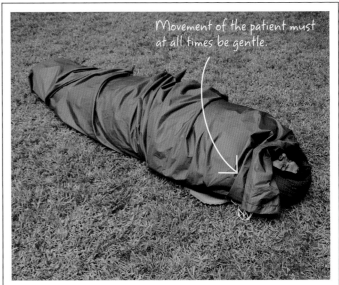

Movement of the patient must at all times be gentle.

- Patients with severe hypothermia have cold heart muscles requiring very gentle handling.

- They need their clothes removed. To maximize gentleness, the clothes should be cut off.

- They need to be bundled in multiple layers of dry material. The final layer should be windproof and waterproof, such as a sheet of plastic. They need to be insulated from the cold ground.

- Movement of such patients is best performed by a team of rescuers who lift the patients slowly and gently.

Supplemental oxygen would be of great benefit to the patient with severe hypothermia. If supplemental oxygen is unavailable, mouth-to-mouth breathing, started when breathing is undetectable or barely detectable, may help keep a severely hypothermic patient alive. Breathe for the patient for five to fifteen minutes before moving.

Gently remove clothing, cutting it away if at all possible. You may, in fact, need to cut it to remove it. Lift the patient gently onto a dry "bed" of insulation. The thicker the insulation, the better for the patient. If snow or rain is falling, take care to keep the insulation as dry as possible. Insulation such as sleeping pads must adequately protect the patient from the ground. Patient and insulation should be enclosed in a layer of material that allows no air or water through, such as a sheet of plastic. The resulting cocoon leaves only the patient's face exposed. Hot water bottles or heat packs may be applied to the patient's chest, but wrap the heat source in dry material first.

Go for help. Do not attempt to move the patient without professional assistance.

Treatment

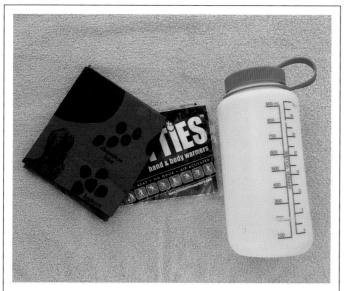

- A severely hypothermic patient will benefit from the application of low-intensity heat sources such as hot water bottles and chemical heat packs.

- These heat sources should not be placed directly on skin but rather wrapped first in a thin layer of mate-rial such as a bandanna. Cold skin burns easily.

- The most critical place to apply the heat source is over the heart.

- Additional heat sources may be applied to the neck and armpits.

Severe Hypothermia Management

- Handle the patient gently.

- Give rescue breaths for five to fifteen minutes before moving.

- Put the patient in a hypothermia wrap.

- Call for help.

PREVENTING HYPOTHERMIA

It is much easier to stay warm than to get warm again

Hypothermia is an entirely preventable problem. Knowledge is the key to prevention. It is more important to stay dry than to stay comfortably warm.

When exposed to cold weather, you need to dress properly. The best cold-weather clothing is made of material that "wicks" sweat away from your body, clothing made of synthetic fibers woven into garments. Wool garments will work because they retain body heat when damp. Cotton is not recommended. Wear clothing in layers instead of wearing bulky garments. Layers can be opened but more importantly removed when you warm up and put back on when you cool off, allowing you to stay dry when exercising.

Stay well hydrated. Avoid thirst. Drink enough fluid—and water is best—to keep your urine colorless or light in color. Avoid alcohol and highly caffeinated beverages.

Stay well fed. Simple carbohydrates, such as candies, are

Dress Appropriately

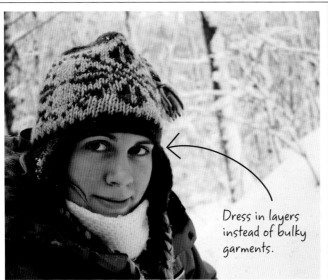

Dress in layers instead of bulky garments.

- Wear clothing that holds in body heat even when wet, clothing made of synthetics or wool.

- Wear clothing in layers that allow you to remove layers when you start to sweat and put layers back on when you start to feel a chill.

- Wear a stocking cap that covers at least your ears and a parka with a hood for further head and neck protection.

- Wear mittens and cold-weather footwear.

Hydration

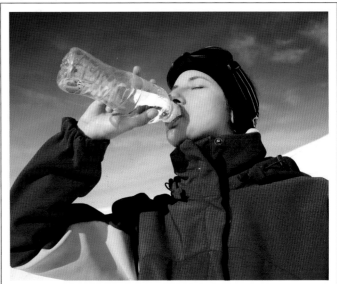

- Heat is carried from warm body parts to cold body parts by your circulating blood. Blood also carries glucose to fuel your muscles as they produce heat.

- You must stay adequately hydrated to maintain an adequate amount of blood volume.

- Although there may be a slight benefit from drinking warm fluids, your body will handle cold fluids well.

- Drink enough to keep your urine clear or at least a light yellow.

more quickly digested into energy than are more complex foods. But complex carbohydrates, such as whole grain foods, are needed for more sustained energy.

Pace yourself when exercising in cold. Avoid overexertion, which results in sweat, fatigue, and loss of stored energy.

Because even mild hypothermia causes a drop in mental acuity, it is usually easier to see and reverse the early stages in someone else than in yourself.

COLD WEATHER

Nutrition

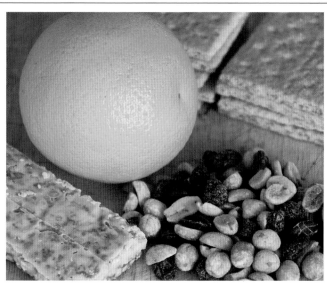

- The food you eat is turned into energy, and heat is produced. The harder you exercise, the more fuel you burn and the more heat you produce.

- Simple carbohydrates, such as sugar-rich foods, are digested the quickest

and turned into heat the quickest.

- You need to snack regularly in cold weather to be sure your internal fires are stoked.

- Carry snacks in an outside pocket of your clothing for quick access.

Pacing

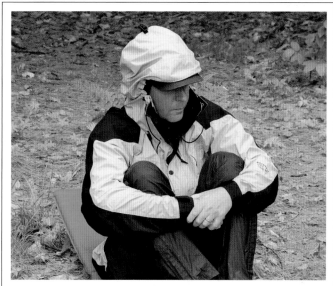

- To prevent hypothermia, it is more important to stay dry than to stay comfortably warm.

- Sweating is the primary source of moisture that collects on your skin and in your clothing.

- Pace yourself when you exercise in cold. Move at a pace that keeps you sweating at a minimum.

- Take rest breaks often, and add layers of clothing while resting to prevent the heat you've generated from being lost to the environment.

FROSTBITE

The depth of the frozen tissue determines the severity of the problem

Frostbite is localized tissue damage caused by freezing, a problem most likely to occur at the extremities of the body: ears, nose, fingers, and toes. It creates a spectrum of injuries depending on how cold the tissue becomes.

Frostbite is progressive, moving from mild to severe if untreated. Superficial frostbite looks pale and feels cold and numb, but the skin is still elastic. Partial thickness frostbite may appear superficial until after warming, when blisters develop. The darker the color of the fluid filling the blisters, the worse the damage. Full thickness frostbite is icy cold, and skin is white and hard.

Damage from frostbite occurs in two phases, the freezing

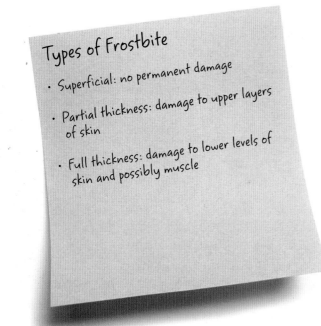

Types of Frostbite

- Superficial: no permanent damage

- Partial thickness: damage to upper layers of skin

- Full thickness: damage to lower levels of skin and possibly muscle

Skin-to-skin Warming

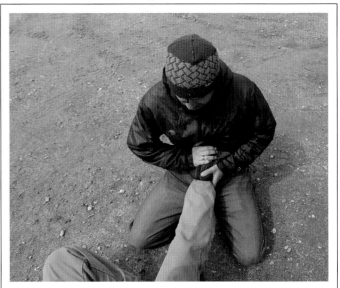

- Superficial frostbite and partial thickness frostbite should be warmed as soon as possible.

- This can be achieved outdoors with passive skin-to-skin warming, placing the frostbitten part against warm areas of your body or against warm areas of another person's body.

- Do *not* massage the injury, and do *not* warm the injury with radiant heat. These actions cause more injury.

- As soon as possible, get out of the cold. It is imperative to prevent refreezing.

phase and the thawing phase. Blood flow decreases during the freezing phase, and ice crystals form in the fluid between cells, drawing fluid out of the cells and dehydrating them. More damage can occur mechanically if the ice crystals rub against each other, a warning to handle frostbitten tissue gently. During the thawing phase, the damaged cells release substances that promote clot formation and vasoconstriction. More damage occurs during the thawing phase than during the freezing phase.

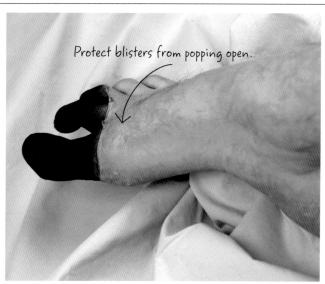

· · · · · · · · · · · · · · · · RED ● LIGHT · · · · · · · · · · · · · ·

Anyone who develops blisters after frozen tissue is warmed needs to be evaluated by a physician—and the sooner, the better. Warning: Blisters will refreeze much faster than normal tissue.

Warm Water

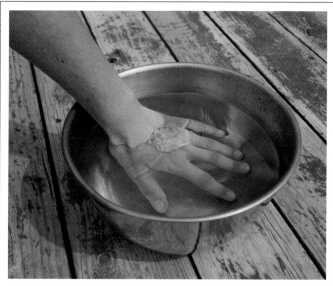

After Warming

Protect blisters from popping open.

- The best warming method for frostbite is to immerse the injury in water warmed to 99–102°F.

- This is best done in a hospital, and it is especially important to get someone with hard-frozen tissue to a hospital as soon as possible.

- If transportation is delayed, start the warming process as soon as you can get warm water.

- You will have to keep adding warm water to the container to keep the water warm enough.

- After warming, the patient typically feels pain. The worse the injury, the greater the pain. The pain can become extreme.

- Aspirin or ibuprofen may help with pain, and both aspirin and ibuprofen are beneficial in reducing the extent of the injury.

- If blisters form and/or the skin develops marked discoloration, the injury may be wrapped loosely in soft material to provide protection.

- Protect the injury from being bumped or otherwise roughly handled.

PREVENTING FROSTBITE
Frostbite develops due to lack of proper preventive steps

As with hypothermia, frostbite is a preventable problem. Predisposing factors related to frostbite include moisture on skin, low ambient temperatures (which must be below freezing for frostbite to occur), high winds (which speed heat loss), dehydration, and poor nutrition.

Wear adequate cold-weather clothing (see "Preventing Hypothermia"), including boots made for winter use. Wearing extra socks in summer boots during winter is not recommended.

Keep all clothing and footwear as dry as possible.

Avoid constricting clothing, especially tight boots. Loose clothing improves circulation, and circulation carries warmth.

Wear mittens instead of gloves. Mittens allow fingers to share warmth, and circulation is better.

Wear a stocking cap that completely covers your ears. In extremes of cold, wear a balaclava to protect your ears and nose.

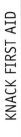

Dress Appropriately

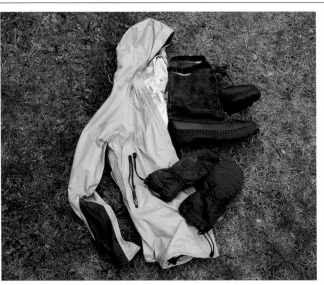

- Avoid tight clothing and footwear in order to promote healthy circulation.

- Mittens allow fingers to share warmth and are looser than gloves, making them overall a better choice.

- Be sure that boots are insu-lated for cold-weather use. Do not put on extra socks inside warm-weather boots, a practice that reduces circulation.

- If your cold-weather clothing prevents heat loss from your body, it will be easier to keep your feet and hands warm.

Hydration and Nutrition

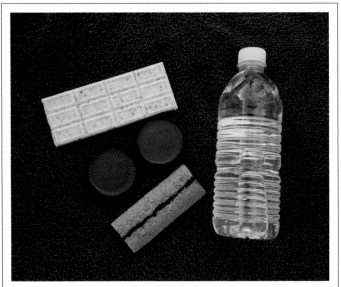

- As with preventing hypothermia, staying well hydrated reduces the chance of cold injury. Carry water, and drink often when outside in cold weather.

- Prior to exposure to cold, eat well to build up energy stores for heat production.

- Simple carbohydrates (sugars) burn quickly and should be kept handy for a quick addition of internal fuel.

- Complex carbohydrates (starches) burn more slowly, and fats burn the slowest of all. Your pre-exposure meal should include both.

Avoid skin contact with cold metal and cold gasoline, both of which could cause frostbite on contact.

Stay well hydrated. Dehydration reduces blood volume, and blood is necessary to maintain warmth in small (and large) body parts.

Maintain a high-calorie diet. Food is fuel burned to create internal warmth.

Watch companions for the early signs of frostbite, including white patches on the face.

When fingers and toes tingle and/or feel painfully cold, stop and warm them immediately. If they go numb, the pain ends, but frostbite is near.

Things to Avoid

Alcohol makes you feel warm but speeds heat loss.

- Alcoholic beverages cause blood vessels to dilate (open up), giving you a feeling of warmth but actually increasing the rate at which you lose heat.

- Nicotine causes blood vessels to constrict (close down), increasing the risk of frostbite to small body parts.

- Strong caffeinated drinks increase the risk of dehydration and therefore increase the risk of frostbite.

- Some medications predispose you to cold injury. Check with your doctor or pharmacist if you are taking drugs.

More Tips

- If your toes hurt, stop and warm them; if they go numb, it might be too late.

- Far from a vehicle or building, carry extra clothing, socks, mittens, and cap.

- If you get wet, change into dry clothing as soon as possible.

NONFREEZING COLD INJURY
Skin does not have to freeze to create the threat of lost toes

Nonfreezing cold injury (NFCI) is a cold-weather emergency resulting from prolonged contact with cold—and usually also with moisture—that causes inadequate circulation with resulting tissue damage. You may have heard it called "trenchfoot" or "immersion foot."

Initially the damaged tissue is cold and pale or mottled in color and possibly swollen. After the tissue warms, pain and itching are the dominant symptoms. The damaged skin may

also look red, swell, and feel unusually hot after warming. Some patients will complain that their foot is numb.

Warm the foot by immersion in water of 99–102 F or by skin-to-skin contact (see "Frostbite"). Dry the foot gently or allow it to air-dry if the air is warm. Keep the foot elevated slightly above the level of the patient's heart. Do not rub the foot or place it near a strong heat source, actions that will likely further damage tissue. Start the patient on a regimen of

Nonfreezing Cold Injury

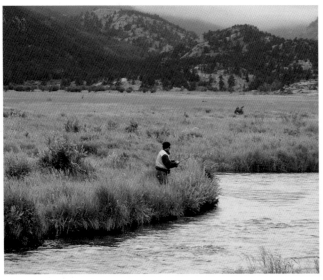

- A medical problem resulting from prolonged exposure to damp, cold, and possibly unsanitary conditions

- It most often occurs when someone is submerged in

seawater or hiking through wet conditions in a cold environment.

- A nonfreezing injury is sometimes referred to as "trench-foot" or "immersion foot."

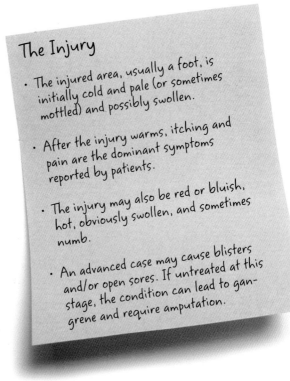

The Injury

- The injured area, usually a foot, is initially cold and pale (or sometimes mottled) and possibly swollen.

- After the injury warms, itching and pain are the dominant symptoms reported by patients.

- The injury may also be red or bluish, hot, obviously swollen, and sometimes numb.

- An advanced case may cause blisters and/or open sores. If untreated at this stage, the condition can lead to gangrene and require amputation.

over-the-counter anti-inflammatory drugs (aspirin or ibuprofen), following the directions on the label, if a doctor cannot soon be found. Remember that it will probably take twenty-four to forty-eight hours before the severity of the damage is fully apparent.

Treatment

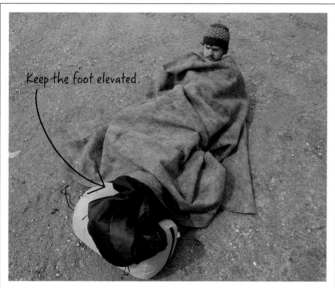

Keep the foot elevated.

Preventing NFCI

- In cold, damp conditions outdoors, dry your feet and put on dry socks twice a day.

- If sleeping outdoors, do not sleep with cold, wet feet.

- Stay well hydrated and well nourished.

- As soon as nonfreezing cold injury is assessed, the foot should be warmed without massage and without exposure to high radiant heat.

- The foot should be kept dry and kept elevated to or above the level of the patient's heart.

- Any constriction of the injury, such as boots, should be avoided, and the area must be kept safe from further injury.

- Pain may be treated with over-the-counter pain-killing drugs.

143

HEAT EXHAUSTION

Although not a serious threat, heat exhaustion makes you feel terrible

"Heat illness" describes a range of problems associated with a rise in air temperature—everything from the fatigue of heat exhaustion to the life threat of heat stroke.

With *heat exhaustion*, the patient has been exercising, sweating out water and salt, and now feels very tired. Skin may appear pale and sweaty or flushed and sweaty, and the patient complains of a headache, perhaps nausea, and sometimes vomiting. Thirst is usual, as is a decreased urine output. Dizziness may strike when the patient stands quickly. An elevated heart rate and respiratory rate are common.

The problem is a volume problem—not enough water inside the patient—and it is typically not serious. Core

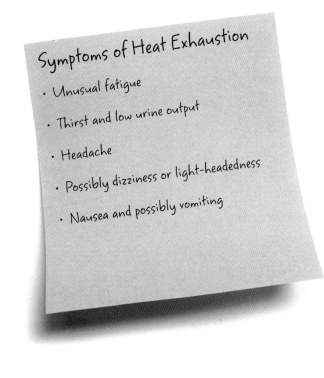

Symptoms of Heat Exhaustion

- Unusual fatigue
- Thirst and low urine output
- Headache
- Possibly dizziness or light-headedness
- Nausea and possibly vomiting

Treatment

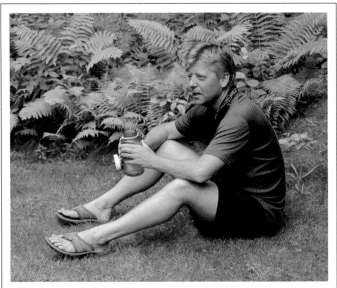

- As the problem suggests, someone suffering from heat exhaustion needs to rest, preferably in a cool, shady spot.

- The patient usually benefits from being fanned, and the addition of wet cotton, such as a bandanna, tied around the neck, increases cooling.

- This person is dehydrated and needs to drink. Water is fine, but if you add a pinch of salt to a quart of water, the patient will usually benefit even more.

- This person may also consume sports drinks to rehydrate.

temperature may have risen a few degrees but more often not at all. The cure is suggested by the name of the condition: Exhaustion calls for rest, preferably in a cool, shady spot. Replace lost fluids by drinking water and lost salt by adding a pinch (just a pinch) to a quart of water or by munching salty snacks. Oral rehydration salts or a sports drink will work. Do *not* use salt tablets—they are too concentrated. To increase the rate of cooling, the patient may be wet down and fanned. A drowsy patient may be allowed to sleep.

Heat Cramps

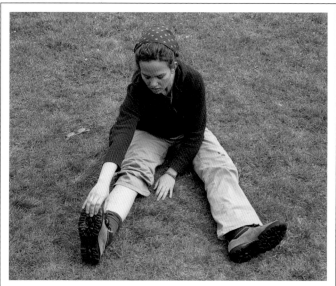

- Heat cramps are sometimes associated with heat exhaustion.

- The cramps are most often in the legs, especially the lower legs, but they may extend up into the abdomen or lower back.

- The cramps are caused by salt depletion, and salt in the fluid being consumed by the patient helps alleviate the problem.

- Heat cramps are eased by gentle stretching of the painful muscles, but aggressive massaging of the muscles is not recommended.

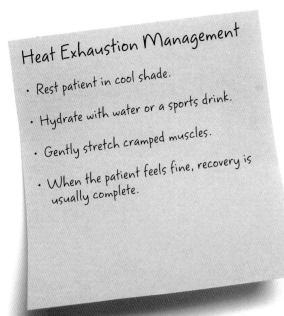

Heat Exhaustion Management

- Rest patient in cool shade.

- Hydrate with water or a sports drink.

- Gently stretch cramped muscles.

- When the patient feels fine, recovery is usually complete.

HEAT STROKE
When the brain gets too hot, death can occur in a short time

Heat stroke occurs when a patient is producing core heat faster than it can be shed. The patient may be overexerting and/or seriously dehydrated, and the core temperature rises to 105 F or more. Disorientation and bizarre personality changes are common signs. Skin turns hot and red and sometimes (but far from always) dry. Look for a fast heart rate, fast breathing, and complaints of a headache.

Heat stroke is a temperature problem. The patient is too hot inside. Once a human brain gets that hot, it is a *true emergency*, and only rapid cooling will save the patient. Take off any heat-retaining clothes, and drench the patient with water. Concentrate cooling efforts on the head and neck. Cold packs may be used on the neck, armpits, groin, and the hands and feet. Fan the patient constantly to increase evaporation. Massage the limbs to encourage cooler blood to return to the core. When, or if, the patient is able to accept

Step 1: Move and Remove

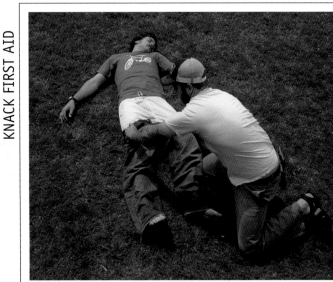

- Heat stroke is an immediate threat to life due to the rising temperature of the patient's brain, and first aid, therefore, must be provided immediately.

- Move the patient quickly to a shady spot, out of the direct rays of the sun.

- Remove all the patient's outer clothing. Clothing retains heat and slows cooling.

- Remove the patient's underwear if it is not cotton. Cotton underwear, once wet, will increase the rate of cooling.

Step 2: Wet

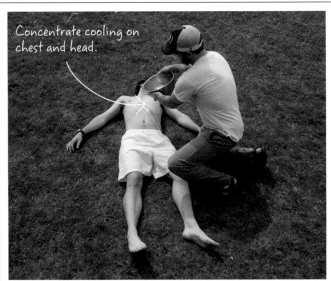

Concentrate cooling on chest and head.

- Cold water will remove heat from the patient faster than any other medium.

- If you can place the patient in a cold stream or lake, do so, but someone must be in the water with the patient to assure that the patient does not drown.

- Without a stream or lake, pour water, the coldest available, onto the patient. If the patient is wearing cotton underclothing, be sure to thoroughly soak the cotton.

- Concentrate your cooling efforts on the chest and head.

and drink cold water, give it. Do *not* give fever-reducing drugs. A careful watch on the patient should be maintained. Relapses are common.

Step 3: Fan

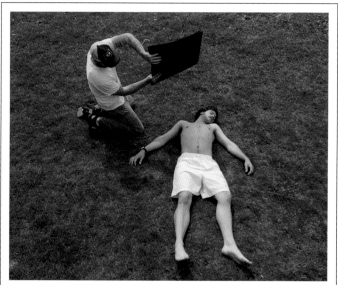

- With a wet patient, moving air will increase the rate of evaporation and therefore increase the rate of cooling.

- If a breeze is blowing, be sure the patient is located in a spot that receives the breeze.

- With or without a breeze, fan the patient aggressively to maximize the cooling rate.

- Use as a fan something that moves a large volume of air so that the patient's skin receives as much "wind" as possible.

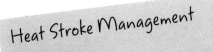

Heat Stroke Management

- Act quickly.

- Move the patient to shade, and remove clothing.

- Wet the patient.

- Fan the patient aggressively.

- Call for help!

HYPONATREMIA

High water intake with low salt intake can create a big problem

You can drink too much water—if you are not eating. Salt loss in sweat exceeding salt intake plus water intake exceeding water loss equals lowered sodium level in the blood. When blood sodium gets too low, you have a case of *hyponatremia*.

Common complaints include headache, weakness, fatigue, light-headedness, muscle cramps, nausea with or without vomiting, sweaty skin, normal core temperature, and normal or slightly elevated pulse and respirations. Sound familiar?

Yes, it sounds like heat exhaustion. But if you treat it like heat exhaustion—just add water—you are harming the hyponatremia patient. More severe symptoms include disorientation, irritability, and combativeness, giving the problem a more common name: water intoxication. Untreated, the ultimate result will be seizures, coma, and death.

Heat-exhausted patients typically have a low output of yellowish urine (urinating every six to eight hours) combined with

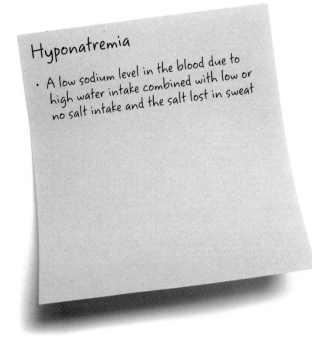

Hyponatremia

- A low sodium level in the blood due to high water intake combined with low or no salt intake and the salt lost in sweat

Treatment: Mild to Moderate

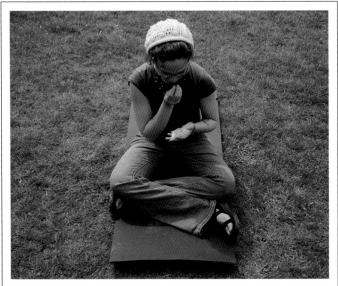

- Because hyponatremia looks like heat exhaustion, be sure of your assessment.

- The hyponatremia patient has been drinking plenty of fluids, has been urinating often, and has not been eating.

- The patient needs to rest,

preferably in a cool, shady spot, but the patient should be given nothing to drink. Sports drinks should be avoided!

- The patient needs a slow intake of salty food until recovery is complete. Once the patient feels fine, the patient has recovered.

thirst. Hyponatremia patients have urinated recently, and the urine was probably clear. Hyponatremia patients claim to have been drinking a lot of water, and they deny thirst.

Patients with mild to moderate symptoms and a normal mental status may be treated by you: rest in shade with no fluid intake and a gradual intake of salty foods. Once a patient develops hunger and thirst combined with normal urine output, the problem is solved.

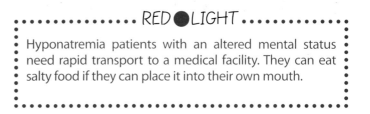

········· RED ● LIGHT ·············

Hyponatremia patients with an altered mental status need rapid transport to a medical facility. They can eat salty food if they can place it into their own mouth.

Treatment: Severe

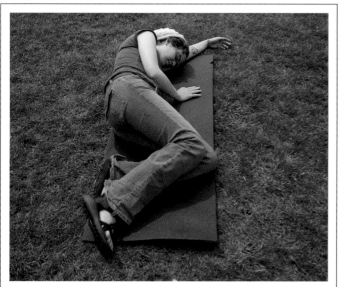

- In addition to the signs and symptoms of mild to moderate hyponatremia, the severe patient will be increasingly disoriented, irritable, and combative.

- Patients who cannot accept salty food from you and place it in their own mouths should not be given food.

- Patients who lapse into unconsciousness should be placed in a stable side position in order to maintain a clear airway.

- Rapid transport to a medical facility is of the utmost importance.

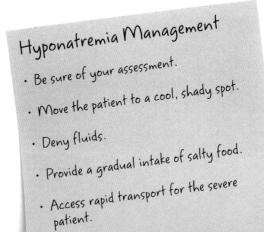

Hyponatremia Management

- Be sure of your assessment.

- Move the patient to a cool, shady spot.

- Deny fluids.

- Provide a gradual intake of salty food.

- Access rapid transport for the severe patient.

HOT WEATHER

149

PREVENTING HEAT ILLNESSES

Taking the proper steps can prevent all heat illnesses

In addition to rising temperatures, other factors increase the risk of heat illnesses: (1) being in high humidity, (2) being overweight, (3) being very young or very old, (4) being unaccustomed to heat, (5) taking certain drugs, such as antihistamines (consult your physician), and (6) being dehydrated (often the most important factor).

The best indication of adequate hydration is urine output that is clear and relatively copious. When exercising in heat, most people need four or more quarts of fluid per day. Water is probably best to drink, and sports drinks are okay. It is practically impossible to drink too much water, unless you are not eating (see "Hyponatremia"). So, munch on lightly salted snacks. Avoid alcohol and caffeinated drinks.

Wear baggy, loosely woven clothing that allows evaporation of sweat. Keep your head covered with a brimmed hat to shade face and neck.

Hydration

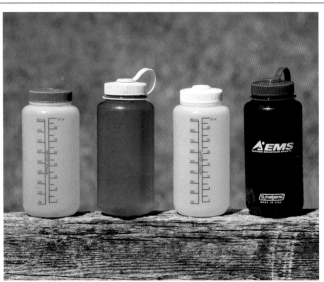

- Anyone who is dehydrated is more likely to suffer problems associated with a hot environment.

- People should be drinking enough water to keep their urine clear or a light yellow, and they should be urinating relatively often.

- Although individuals vary, most people will do well to drink four quarts of water a day in hot weather.

- Drinks high in caffeine and alcoholic beverages should be avoided when your goal is adequate hydration.

Clothing

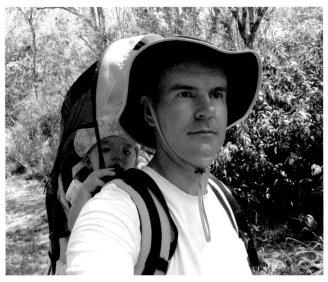

- To reduce heat stress, wear clothing that fits loosely and that is loosely woven. This type of clothing allows air to reach your skin, encouraging evaporation and increasing cooling.

- Light-colored clothing reflects heat (a plus), and dark-colored clothing absorbs heat (a minus).

- Cotton clothing will retain moisture and help you stay cool.

- You need a hat to help keep your head cool. A brim of 3 inches or more will adequately shade your face.

Fit people typically adjust to heat better than the nonfit. But you still need to allow time for acclimatization when you are new to a hot environment. Go slow the first few days, and avoid being exposed to heat during the hottest times of day. If you are exercising in heat, take rest breaks often, in shade, and cool yourself with water-soaked clothing, such as a cotton T-shirt.

ZOOM

To aid in prevention, keep water handy in a pack or automobile, and drink as an act of discipline and not necessarily only when you feel thirsty.

Snacks

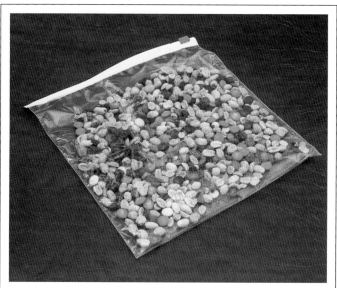

- There is no risk from drinking too much water as long as you are snacking regularly.

- The snacks do not need to be excessively high in salt content, but they do need to contain salt.

- Most sports drinks contain sodium, perhaps enough to be substituted for salty foods, but read the label on the drink to be sure.

- You will get enough sodium if you put a pinch of salt into a quart bottle of water.

More Tips

- When it's hot, limit your exposure to heat to early and late in the day.

- When new to a hot environment, it takes ten to fourteen days to acclimatize to the heat.

- The very young and the elderly are more susceptible to heat stress.

HOT WEATHER

LIGHTNING
Lightning causes injuries and deaths in several ways

The awesome power of a lightning strike may produce several types of patients, many of them seriously injured and in need of a first-aid provider.

The most common cause of death is cardiac arrest, the result of the current of electricity. After a lightning strike, assess and treat first those patients who appear dead—they might be recoverable. The patients may respond to CPR (see "Adult CPR").

Sometimes the heart stops and then starts up again, but breathing does not. This patient is likely to respond to rescue breathing (see "Rescue Breathing").

A lightning strike is loud and bright, and a nearby strike may cause complaints of ringing in the ears or loss of hearing. Temporary loss of sight is not unusual. These patients often recover in time, but an evaluation by a physician is by far the best bet.

Respiratory and Cardiac Arrest

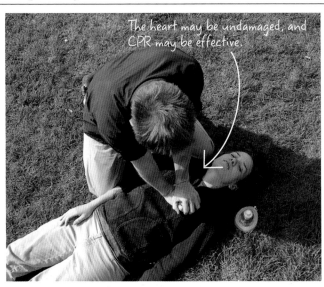

The heart may be undamaged, and CPR may be effective.

- Direct strikes of lightning to humans are rare, but the electrical charge can reach people by "splashing" off a nearby object, by running down a conductor (such as a fence), or by moving through ground current.

- The electrical charge can cause respiratory and cardiac arrest in someone.

- Patients in respiratory arrest often respond only to rescue breathing.

- Although cardiac arrest is always a tremendously serious event, the patient may respond to CPR done well.

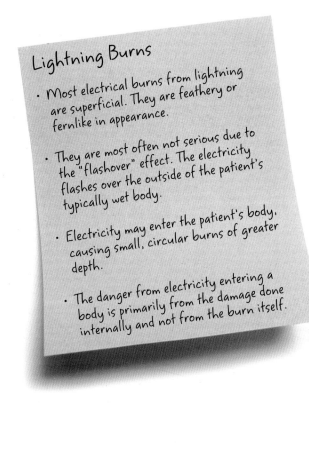

Lightning Burns

- Most electrical burns from lightning are superficial. They are feathery or fernlike in appearance.

- They are most often not serious due to the "flashover" effect. The electricity flashes over the outside of the patient's typically wet body.

- Electricity may enter the patient's body, causing small, circular burns of greater depth.

- The danger from electricity entering a body is primarily from the damage done internally and not from the burn itself.

Serious burns from lightning are unusual, but superficial, feathery, fernlike, or linear burns are common (see "Burns").

Lightning explodes the air, and the blast can toss people around and into objects, causing all types of injuries, including fractures, dislocations, wounds, head injuries, and spine injuries. Check the patient thoroughly.

Eye and Ear Injuries

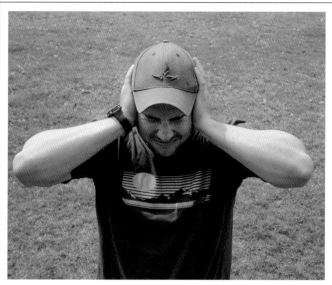

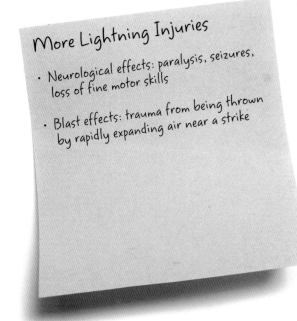

More Lightning Injuries

- Neurological effects: paralysis, seizures, loss of fine motor skills

- Blast effects: trauma from being thrown by rapidly expanding air near a strike

- Temporary blindness from a lightning strike is common due to the intensity of the light from lightning and the shock waves passing through the air near a strike.

- If electricity enters the eyes, nerve damage can occur, and blindness can be permanent.

- Temporary deafness is also common and due to the loud noise and the accompanying shock waves.

- The noise may rupture eardrums and cause nerve damage to the ears.

LIGHTNING SAFETY

Although lightning has an unpredictable aspect, you can avoid almost all injuries

Lightning safety involves understanding the nature of lightning and planning ahead.

You need to know local weather patterns. Thunderstorms bring lightning, and storms, in general, tend to roll in quickly in the afternoon of summer months.

Watch the sky, and plot storms. When the flash of lightning precedes the boom of thunder by five seconds, the storm is approximately 1 mile away. Although rarely lightning has been known to reach out 10 miles ahead of a storm, you are most often safe if you find shelter or a safe spot before the storm is 6 miles away—when the flash precedes the boom by thirty seconds.

Avoid Open Spaces

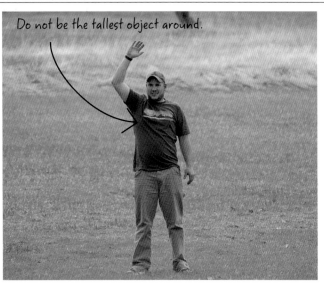

Do not be the tallest object around.

- Many people injured by lightning are caught in open spaces during a storm.

- They are injured because they are the tallest object around, and lightning often strikes the tallest object. Lightning tends to take the shortest route from a cloud to a target.

- Golfers are at risk on open fairways and greens.

- Anglers are at risk when fishing from open shorelines and from boats on open bodies of water.

Avoid Tall Objects

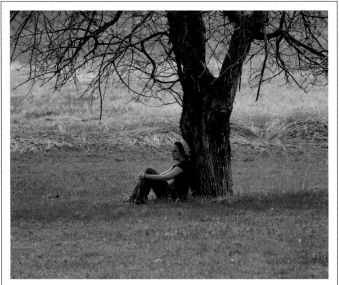

- The electrical charge of lightning can "splash" after hitting tall objects, causing injury to someone standing near a tall object.

- Move well away from isolated tall trees, power poles, high points of land, or anything obviously higher than other objects in the area.

- Seek cover in stands of trees of uniform height, but avoid contact with a tree.

- Seek cover in low, rolling hills, but do not stand at the top of a low hill.

What is a safe spot? Avoid high places, high objects, open places, low places, shallow caves, overhangs, places obviously struck in the past, and long conductors (such as fences). Metal does not attract lightning, but it conducts it extremely well. Stay well away from metal. Open bodies of water, especially the shoreline, are dangerous. Try to get boats to shore, and move, if possible, at least 200 feet from shore. Seek uniform cover such as low rolling hills or trees of about the same size, but do not lean against a tree. Generally safe are deep, dry caves, buildings (away from windows and walls), and cars or trucks with the windows rolled up.

If you are outside, assume a safe position. Squat or sit in a tight position, arms wrapped around legs, on insulating material such as a sleeping pad. Do not lie down.

If you are with a group, spread people out, but try to keep everyone in sight. You don't want a lightning strike to leave no one able to help.

If you are camping, choose a campsite that meets the safety requirements.

Avoid Conductors

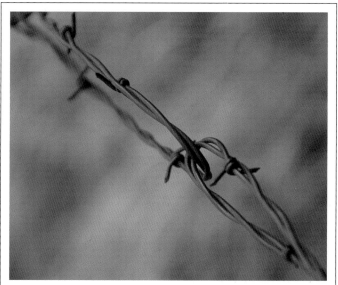

- The electrical charge of lightning will travel rapidly, dangerously, and for a long way along material that easily conducts electricity.

- During storms, avoid contact with wire fences, wires, pipes, and railroad tracks. Even wet ropes will conduct electricity.

- Metal does not attract lightning, but it is an especially good conductor. Avoid contact with any metal, even when you are inside a building.

- If you are in a vehicle, keep the windows up and avoid contact with metal parts.

More Safety Tips

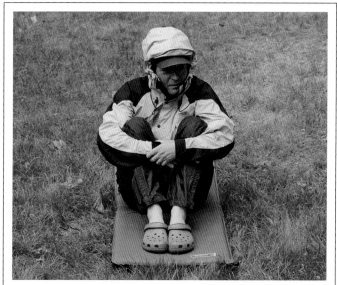

- If you are outside, do not lie down. Sit in a tight position to minimize your contact with the ground, preferably on some type of insulating material.

- If you seek shelter in a cave, the cave must be dry to be safe.

- If rain can reach underneath an overhanging rock, so can lightning.

- If you are in a building, avoid the windows and fireplaces, and do not use a telephone.

155

DROWNING

Those who have died from being submerged in water may still be viable

At this writing, drowning (suffocation from water filling the lungs) is the third-leading cause of accidental death in the United States. Many of those who have died could have been saved with proper emergency care.

People who drown typically panic and struggle fiercely to reach the surface of the water they are in. They also fight against the need to breathe. When the need to breathe wins, they inhale water, and loss of consciousness soon follows. It is not long before respiratory arrest and then cardiac arrest.

As soon as you have access to the patient, check for breathing (see "Check for Breathing"). If you can't detect breathing, start rescue breathing (see "Rescue Breathing"). Rescue

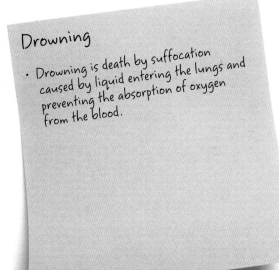

Drowning

- Drowning is death by suffocation caused by liquid entering the lungs and preventing the absorption of oxygen from the blood.

Rescue Breathing

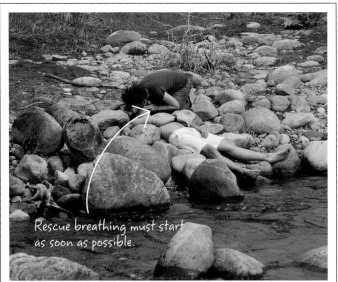

Rescue breathing must start as soon as possible.

- Start rescue breathing for a drowned person as soon as possible, even while the person is still in water if you are stable (such as standing in shallow water).

- Do not waste time trying to remove water from the lungs—it does not work.

- The person may vomit, so be ready to roll the person to remove vomitus from the airway.

- If vomiting does occur, rescue breathing must resume as soon as the airway is cleared.

breathing can sometimes be started in shallow water prior to completely removing the patient from the water.

Do not attempt to remove water from the lungs with abdominal thrusts or any other method. You are wasting time that could be used in rescue breathing.

As soon as the patient is on a firm surface, check for a pulse and other signs of circulation (see "Adult CPR"). In the absence of a pulse, start CPR.

CPR

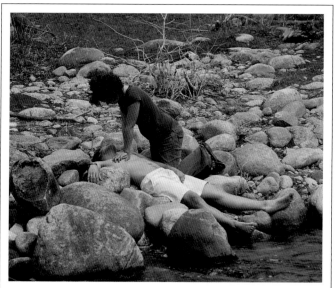

- For a drowned person, CPR must be initiated as soon as possible. The sooner it is started, the greater the chance of success.

- The patient must be on a firm surface for CPR to be effective.

- CPR is well defined, and

CPR for a drowned person is exactly the same as for any other cause of cardiac arrest.

- Respiratory problems are common after successful resuscitation. The onset is usually within six hours but may be delayed for twenty-four to seventy-two hours.

Submerged Victim Management

- Call 911.

- Remove the patient from the water without endangering yourself.

- Start rescue breathing as soon as possible.

- Start CPR if necessary.

DROWNING, ALTITUDE

PREVENTING DROWNING

Thousands of drowning deaths every year could have been prevented

Most people who have drowned have one thing in common: They did *not* intend to be in the water but instead planned to stay in the boat or on shore.

Many of these people were also nonswimmers. People involved in water-based activities should know how to swim.

And most of these people were not wearing personal flotation devices (PFDs). Life jackets save lives.

Estimates vary, but some experts guess that more than half of all drowned victims had alcohol or another mind-altering substance in their systems.

The loss of coordination that soon follows immersion in icy

Know Your Ability

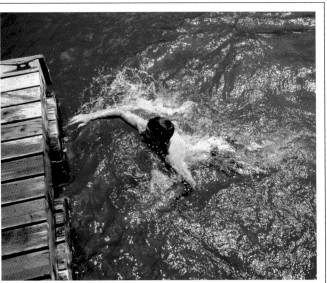

- Learn to swim, and be honest about your ability to swim.

- Until you are a strong swimmer, do not swim where you cannot touch the bottom with your feet.

- Remember that cold water and/or strong currents greatly impair your ability to swim. If you are caught in strong current, swim at an angle across and with the current instead of fighting against the current.

- Swim parallel to shore instead of out into deeper water.

Follow the Rules

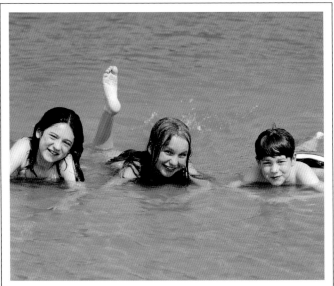

- Never swim alone.

- Never swim after ingesting an alcoholic beverage or any other mind-altering substance.

- Never dive head-first into water unless you have been trained to dive. And never dive into water where you cannot see the bottom unless you know for sure that the water is deep and free of underwater obstacles.

- Never leave children unattended near water. At least one person watching the children must be able to perform a rescue.

water is another factor in why people drown.

When a victim is struggling in the water, fighting to stay alive (see "Drowning"), the risk to a rescuer is great. Here is the appropriate order of events in getting someone out of the water: Reach, throw, row, tow. Reach with your hand or foot or with a long object, from a secure position. Throw the person something that floats. Row or paddle to the person in a stable watercraft. Or throw out a line, and pull the person to safety.

·············· RED ● LIGHT ··············

Do not swim out to save a drowning person unless you are highly trained and willing to risk your life. Fear and panic lend incredible strength to the victim.

PFDs

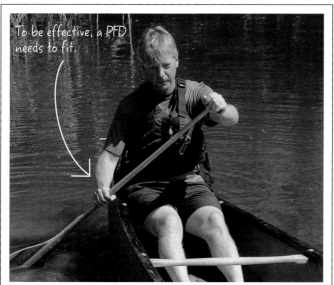

To be effective, a PFD needs to fit.

- Personal flotation devices must be Coast Guard approved, in serviceable condition, and the proper size for the wearer.

- You can slip out of a PFD that is too large for you and a PFD that is too small for you to secure properly.

- Coast Guard–approved PFDs come in five types, and your type should be matched to the conditions you might face.

- PFDs should be worn at all times on small vessels and stored for immediate access on larger vessels.

More Tips

- Do not wade in rapidly moving water that rises above your knees.

- Do not wade in rapidly moving water with a rocky bottom that could entrap your foot.

- Do not swim in rivers unless you have scouted ahead for dangers.

DROWNING, ALTITUDE

159

ACUTE MOUNTAIN SICKNESS

With recent altitude gain, almost everyone experiences a headache

As the altitude above sea level increases, the amount of oxygen available to be inhaled with each breath decreases. This can lead to *hypoxia*, insufficient oxygen in the blood for normal cell function, and when hypoxia affects the cells of the brain and/or lungs, the problems associated with higher altitudes range from mildly annoying to life-threatening.

The most common and least serious form of altitude illness is *acute mountain sickness* (AMS), the first stage of problems associated with the brain. The symptoms can show up in as little as an hour after the patient arrives at a higher altitude, but usually six to ten hours pass before complaints begin.

The symptoms are nonspecific, which means they don't necessarily indicate AMS, and that makes assessment sometimes problematic. But if the patient recently arrived at 8,000 feet or more of elevation, AMS should be your first guess.

Ninety percent or more of patients will complain of a

Symptoms of Acute Mountain Sickness

- Headache
- Nausea and perhaps vomiting
- Loss of appetite
- Insomnia
- Unusual fatigue
- Lassitude (lethargy, sluggishness)

AMS 1

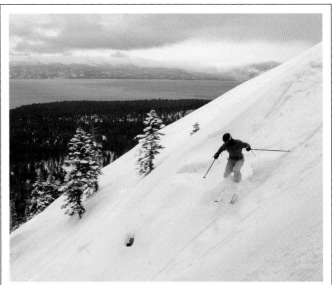

- As you go higher in altitude, the air pressure goes down, and there is less oxygen in every breath of air you inhale. The air is "thinner."

- About 90 percent of people who have recently arrived at an altitude of 8,000 feet or more, such as those on skiing vacations, often com-plain of a headache.

- The most common cause of the headache is acute mountain sickness.

- Acute mountain sickness is not physiologically damaging, but, if ignored, it could progress to life-threatening challenges.

headache. They may also complain of nausea, perhaps with vomiting, loss of normal appetite, inability to sleep well, unusual weariness, exhaustion, or fatigue, and light-headedness.

AMS 2

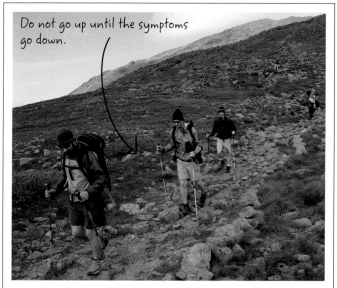

Do not go up until the symptoms go down.

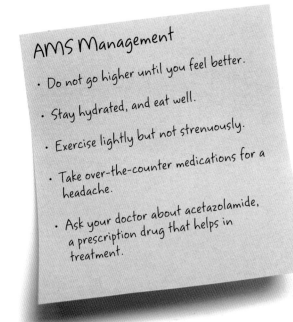

AMS Management

- Do not go higher until you feel better.
- Stay hydrated, and eat well.
- Exercise lightly but not strenuously.
- Take over-the-counter medications for a headache.
- Ask your doctor about acetazolamide, a prescription drug that helps in treatment.

- The signs and symptoms of AMS can show up in as little as an hour after arriving at a higher altitude, but usually it takes an average of six to ten hours before complaints begin.

- Age is not a factor in whether higher altitudes affect you.

- Neither is fitness a factor in whether higher altitudes affect you.

- If you suffered AMS in the past, you are more likely to suffer it again on future trips to higher altitudes.

H.A.C.E.

High altitude cerebral edema is a potentially fatal illness of the brain

A serious threat to the brain associated with higher elevations is high altitude cerebral edema (H.A.C.E.). H.A.C.E. involves fluid leaking from capillaries in the brain and collecting to the point where pressure increases on the brain. The pressure can increase until death is the end result, and quick, proper action by you can prevent it.

H.A.C.E. develops progressively over hours to days. A patient assessed with AMS (see "Acute Mountain Sickness")

who continues to worsen may be headed toward H.A.C.E. Early assessment and treatment provide the patient the best chance of complete recovery.

A terrible headache, perhaps described as the worst the patient has ever experienced, may indicate H.A.C.E. But not all H.A.C.E. patients complain of severe headache.

Be especially aware of *ataxia*, a loss of muscular control leading to difficulty in maintaining balance. You can test

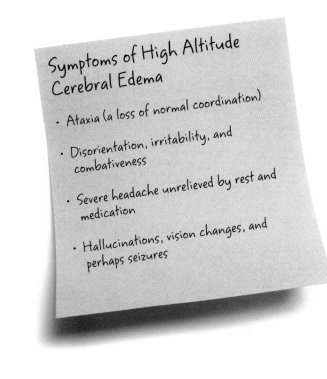

Symptoms of High Altitude Cerebral Edema

- Ataxia (a loss of normal coordination)

- Disorientation, irritability, and combativeness

- Severe headache unrelieved by rest and medication

- Hallucinations, vision changes, and perhaps seizures

H.A.C.E.

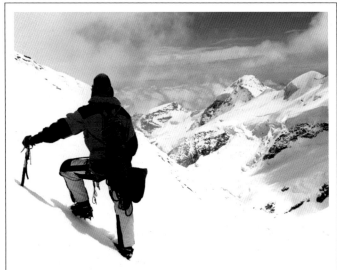

- H.A.C.E. is unusual below 12,000 feet in elevation, but it has been documented at lower elevations.

- It is caused by fluid leaking out of blood vessels and accumulating in the brain, fluid that puts life-threatening pressure on the brain.

- H.A.C.E. is evidenced by the signs and symptoms of acute mountain sickness (AMS) with the addition of ataxia and changes in mental status.

- It is the least common but the most deadly of altitude illnesses.

for early ataxia by asking the patient to walk a straight line on the ground, touching heel to toe. Ataxic people cannot walk the line. A persistent stumbling gait is a sign of more advanced ataxia.

Watch also for alterations in the patient's mental status. H.A.C.E. typically causes disorientation, irritability, and combativeness. Patients may also suffer significant personality changes and hallucinations. You will probably at some point notice sluggishness or drowsiness in the patient. Seizures are possible but not common.

Treatment

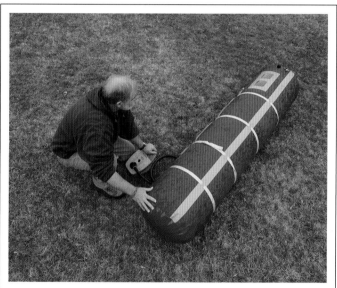

- Descent is the highest priority in the treatment of H.A.C.E. A descent in elevation of 2,000 to 4,000 feet can be life-saving.

- A Gamow bag (pictured) is a portable hyperbaric (high-pressure) chamber that simulates descent for a patient who cannot descend, a patient who cannot walk, and a patient for whom there is no transportation.

- Supplemental oxygen will benefit the patient.

- Drugs proven helpful in the treatment of H.A.C.E. are acetazolamide and dexamethasone.

Anyone assessed with H.A.C.E. needs to be evaluated by a physician. The speed of the need is relative to the intensity of the signs and symptoms.

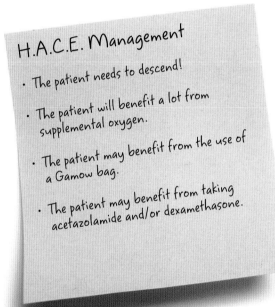

H.A.C.E. Management

- The patient needs to descend!

- The patient will benefit a lot from supplemental oxygen.

- The patient may benefit from the use of a Gamow bag.

- The patient may benefit from taking acetazolamide and/or dexamethasone.

DROWNING, ALTITUDE

163

H.A.P.E.

High altitude pulmonary edema is a potentially fatal illness of the lungs

The most common form of severe altitude illness is high altitude pulmonary edema (H.A.P.E.), in which fluid collects in the lungs, preventing adequate breathing. If enough fluid collects, the patient essentially drowns. Unlike most cases of cerebral edema (see "H.A.C.E."), H.A.P.E. sufferers may recover in the field with proper care.

Indications of H.A.P.E. most often appear during the second night, while the patient is at rest, after that individual reaches a specific high altitude. After four days at a given altitude, H.A.P.E. is unusual. The earliest signs of H.A.P.E. are a decreased ability to exercise and a dry cough. Patients complain of shortness of breath even when they are at rest. As

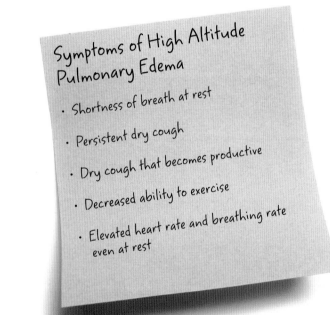

Symptoms of High Altitude Pulmonary Edema

- Shortness of breath at rest

- Persistent dry cough

- Dry cough that becomes productive

- Decreased ability to exercise

- Elevated heart rate and breathing rate even at rest

H.A.P.E. 1

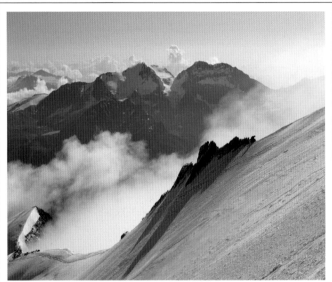

- Fluid leaks out of capillaries in the lungs and collects in the air spaces, making breathing increasingly difficult.

- It is unusual below 8,000 feet of elevation, but it has been seen in patients below 8,000 feet.

- It shows up most often on the second night during sleep after a rapid gain in altitude. It is unusual after four days at a given altitude.

- It is the most common cause of death from altitude illness.

fluid in the lungs increases in volume, later in the progress of the illness, coughing becomes productive, eventually producing frothy sputum that may appear pink with blood. And you may hear gurgling sounds as the patient breathes. The complaint of chest pain is common. As with H.A.C.E., descent is critical if your assessment is H.A.P.E. Descent should be as immediate as possible. If the patient descends under his or her own power, descent should not overexert the patient. Overexertion may exacerbate the problem. If supplemental oxygen is available, the patient will benefit greatly from a high flow.

H.A.P.E. 2

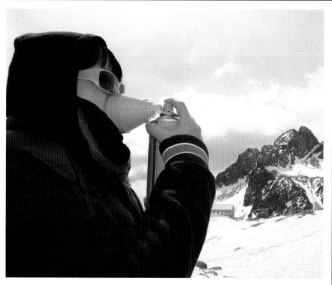

- H.A.P.E. is more common in people who gain altitude quickly than in people who gain altitude slowly.

- It is not known why some people seem predisposed to H.A.P.E. and some do not. Genetic factors may be involved.

- People who have recently had an upper respiratory infection may be more likely to suffer H.A.P.E.

- H.A.P.E. strikes regardless of age, gender, level of physical fitness, diet, or hydration status.

YELLOW LIGHT

Patients who recover from H.A.P.E., usually the result of descent, are not in immediate need of further medical care. But they should be evaluated by a physician when it becomes possible.

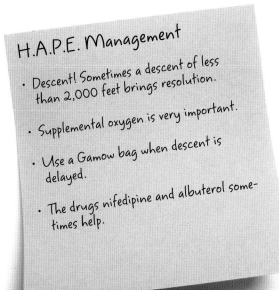

H.A.P.E. Management

- Descent! Sometimes a descent of less than 2,000 feet brings resolution.

- Supplemental oxygen is very important.

- Use a Gamow bag when descent is delayed.

- The drugs nifedipine and albuterol sometimes help.

PREVENTING ALTITUDE ILLNESSES

A few steps in the right direction will prevent most altitude illnesses

Almost everyone will adjust physiologically (acclimatize) to higher altitudes if given enough time. Acclimatization, in other words, usually prevents serious illness.

Above 10,000 feet elevation, most people should gain no more than 1,000–1,500 feet of sleeping altitude for every twenty-four hours. That means they can gain more than 1,500 feet while exercising, but at bedtime they should fall asleep no more than 1,000–1,500 feet higher than the night before.

Adequate water intake may or may not prevent altitude illnesses, but it is essential to maximize acclimatization. Enough water should be consumed daily to keep urine output clear and copious. Eating enough calories is necessary for the energy to exercise and to acclimatize. Carbohydrates require less oxygen to be metabolized, and a high-carb diet may help prevent illnesses but probably not unless the ascent reaches beyond 16,000–17,000 feet elevation.

Acclimatization

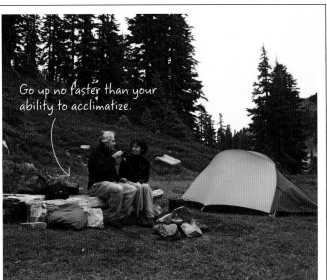

Go up no faster than your ability to acclimatize.

- Acclimatization to altitude is the physiological process of adjusting to "thin air."

- Staging the rate at which you gain altitude will allow your body time to acclimatize.

- If you travel rapidly to an elevation of 10,000 feet or more, take two or three days to rest, and exercise lightly before getting involved in periods of hard exercise.

- Above 10,000 feet, sleep each night at no more than 1,000–1,500 feet higher than the night before.

Prevention Tips

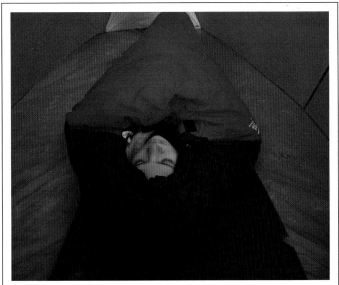

- Do not take sleeping pills. They lower the respiratory drive, making you more susceptible to altitude illness.

- Avoid sedatives and narcotics that suppress the respiratory drive. But if you are taking drugs prescribed by a doctor, keep taking them at altitude.

- Avoid alcoholic beverages, at least until you are acclimatized to a specific altitude.

- Eat well and stay well hydrated. Eating and drinking may not prevent altitude illnesses, but they support the physiological processes involved in acclimatization.

Respiratory depressants, such as sleeping pills and alcohol, should be avoided, especially during the first two or three days at a specific altitude. A doctor may prescribe acetazolamide or dexamethasone for those intolerant of acetazolamide. Both drugs are inarguably effective in reducing the incidence of AMS—but not H.A.C.E. or H.A.P.E.

Acetazolamide

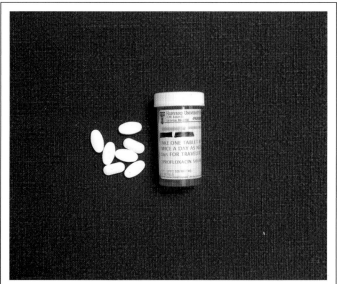

More Tips

- Plan longer vacations, giving yourself acclimatization time.

- Carbohydrates are digested more easily at higher elevations.

- Intentionally take periodic deep breaths.

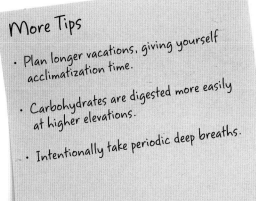

- Acetazolamide is a prescription drug that aids in acclimatization for more than 70 percent of the people who take it.

- The recommended dose for prevention is one-half the dose recommended for the treatment of some altitude illnesses.

- Some people report a side effect of tingling or numbness in the fingers, toes, and mouth. This is harmless.

- Acetazolamide is a diuretic, increasing fluid loss, so special attention must be given to staying well hydrated.

DROWNING, ALTITUDE

MOSQUITOES

In addition to being a nuisance, some mosquitoes carry diseases to humans

Although mosquitoes aggressively pass devastating diseases worldwide, currently only West Nile virus poses a threat in the United States, and that threat is so far minimal.

You can apply an ice pack to minimize the swelling and itching in the first few minutes after a bite, or use an anti-itching product.

Prevention of mosquito bites (and the bites of other small insects) is most easily handled with a repellent. The most effective repellent is DEET, and a concentration of 30 percent, applied to skin, is all that is needed. Higher concentrations last longer but do not increase repellency. DEET should be washed off skin as soon as possible after exposure to insects

Mosquitoes

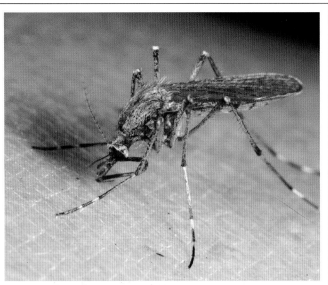

- Worldwide, mosquitoes have a greater impact on humans than any other form of life due to the many diseases they carry and pass to humans.

- Experts estimate that mosquitoes will cause disease in more than 700 million people on this planet in the next year alone.

- Although on the rise, mosquito-borne diseases in the United States are not usual. The most common disease is West Nile virus.

- Mosquitoes in the United States are primarily a nuisance.

Protection

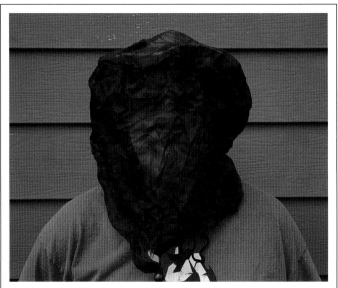

- Head nets prevent mosquitoes from reaching your head and neck. Wear one with a brimmed hat to keep the net off your face.

- Wear clothing thick enough, baggy enough, or tightly woven enough to prevent a mosquito's biting apparatus from reaching your skin.

- Wear long-sleeved shirts and long pants to reduce exposure of skin to mosquitoes.

- When exposed at night, sleep under mosquito netting or inside a tent with mosquito netting covering the door and windows.

has passed. DEET may be applied to clothing, such as collars, cuffs, and hats, in order to repel insects. Permethrin is a potent insect neurotoxin, currently synthesized for human use as an insect repellent, that is applied to clothing or gear such as tents. It should *not* be applied to human skin. After many tests, the experts agree it apparently does no harm to humans, but it quickly loses its efficacy when applied to skin. A third repellent, lemon eucalyptus oil, keeps insects off as effectively as about an 8 percent concentration of DEET.

Repellents

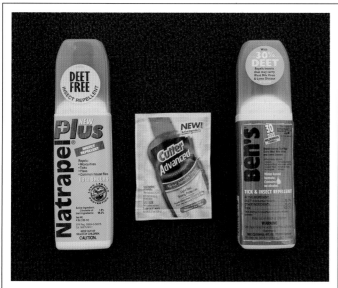

- Products containing DEET repel mosquitoes best. Concentrations higher than 30 percent do not provide more protection, but the protection lasts longer, requiring fewer reapplications.

- DEET should not be applied to skin opened by wounds or irritation, and it should be washed off after exposure has ended. DEET may cause deterioration of plastic, including nylon clothing.

- Other effective repellents include picaridin and lemon eucalyptus oil. Permethrin, applied to clothing, kills mosquitoes before they bite and is harmless to humans.

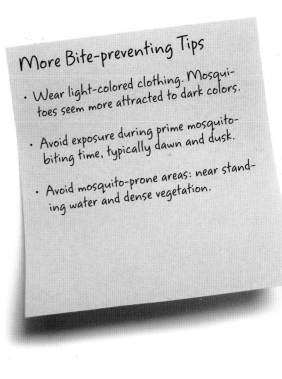

More Bite-preventing Tips

- Wear light-colored clothing. Mosquitoes seem more attracted to dark colors.

- Avoid exposure during prime mosquito-biting time, typically dawn and dusk.

- Avoid mosquito-prone areas: near standing water and dense vegetation.

BITES & STINGS

TICKS

In the United States, ticks pass more diseases to humans than do mosquitoes

A relative of the spider, the tick crawls around on its unsuspecting host on eight tiny legs, looking for the right spot to settle down. It may search for hours. With specialized pincer-like organs, it digs a small wound in its host. Into the wound goes a feeding apparatus, and its relatively powerful sucking mechanism allows the tick to feed on the blood of the host.

Anchored firmly in the wound, it feeds for an average of two to five days, sometimes longer, depending on the species, and drops off weighing hundreds of times more than when it first arrived. In the host it often leaves a reminder of its visit—disease-causing microorganisms. In the United States, ticks pass far more diseases to humans than do mosquitoes.

Tick-borne Diseases in the United States

- Lyme disease
- Rocky Mountain spotted fever
- Colorado tick fever
- Relapsing fever
- Babesiosis
- Tularemia
- Ehrlichiosis

Ticks

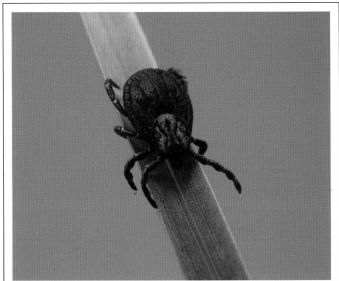

- In the United States, ticks pass more diseases to humans than mosquitoes do.

- Ticks typically crawl over your body for several hours before choosing a site to feed.

- Ticks attach themselves painlessly with a feeding apparatus that allows them to suck blood. They usually feed for several days.

- If they are carrying germs, they do not release the germs all at once but slowly over the days they feed.

Quick tick removal is necessary to reduce the chance of disease transmission. A pair of tweezers should be in your first-aid kit. If the tweezers are fine-pointed, all the better. Grasp the tick near the skin, perpendicular to the longitudinal axis of its body, and pull out gently. No twisting, yanking, or squeezing. After the tick is out, scrub the area gently with alcohol, an antibiotic ointment, or soap and water. Save the tick if you would like to have it checked for disease.

Tick Removal

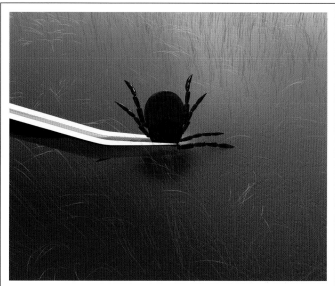

- Ticks found before they have attached have not yet passed germs to you.

- Perform twice-daily tick checks, and remove all embedded ticks as soon as possible.

- Using sharp-tipped tweezers, grasp the tick perpendicular to the long axis of the tick's body and at skin line. Do not squeeze the tick during removal.

- Pull the tick gently straight out without twisting or jerking. You may save the tick's body for a lab test later if you get sick.

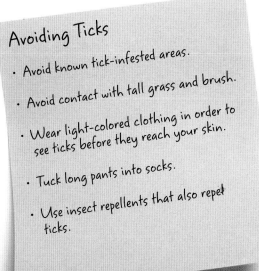

Avoiding Ticks

- Avoid known tick-infested areas.

- Avoid contact with tall grass and brush.

- Wear light-colored clothing in order to see ticks before they reach your skin.

- Tuck long pants into socks.

- Use insect repellents that also repel ticks.

SNAKES

Thousands of bites every year in the United States produce few fatalities

Precise information is lacking, but venomous snakes may bite humans eight thousand to nine thousand times in the United States during the next year. With proper care, these bites will rarely cause death. The snakes to beware are the pit vipers (rattlesnakes, copperheads, and water moccasins) and, far less common, coral snakes. These snakes bite humans when they feel threatened. Most bites occur when a snake is handled or inadvertently stepped on or cornered.

One out of every four or five pit viper bites is "dry"—the snake does not inject venom. Mild envenomations hurt, swell, and turn black and blue—within thirty minutes. Moderate envenomations add swelling that moves up the arm

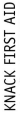

Rattlesnakes

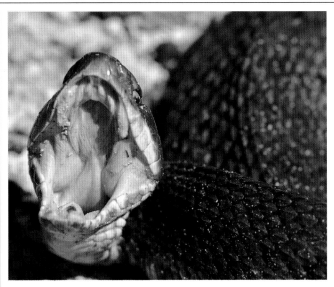

- There are at least thirty-four species and subspecies of pit vipers in the United States.

- All rattlesnakes are pit vipers, with a heat-sensitive pit between their nostrils and their eyes and two hinged, needle-sharp, retractable fangs through which they inject their venom.

- Their venom-injection system is very sophisticated, allowing pit vipers to control the amount of venom they inject.

- One out of every four or five pit viper bites does not involve the injection of venom.

Water Moccasins

- Water moccasins (or cottonmouths) are thick-bodied pit vipers that do not have rattles.

- The world's only semi-aquatic vipers, they are usually found in or near water. They are excellent swimmers in both still and moving water.

- Like all pit vipers, they have a characteristically triangular head obviously distinct from the neck and catlike pupils.

- These snakes will often stand their ground with mouths open, revealing the white lining of their mouths.

or leg toward the heart. Bloody blisters are common, as are weakness, nausea, and perhaps vomiting. Sometimes patients report a "rubbery" taste in their mouths. A severe envenomation might add big jumps in pulse rates and breathing rates, profound swelling, blurred vision, headache, light-headedness, sweating, and chills. Death is possible, most often from respiratory or circulatory collapse.

With coral snakes, envenomation ranges from the mild end, with localized swelling, nausea, and vomiting, to the severe end, with dizziness, weakness, and respiratory difficulty.

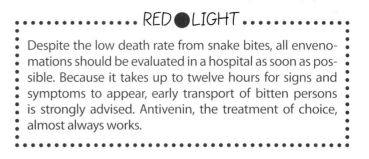

············· RED ● LIGHT ·············

Despite the low death rate from snake bites, all envenomations should be evaluated in a hospital as soon as possible. Because it takes up to twelve hours for signs and symptoms to appear, early transport of bitten persons is strongly advised. Antivenin, the treatment of choice, almost always works.

Copperheads

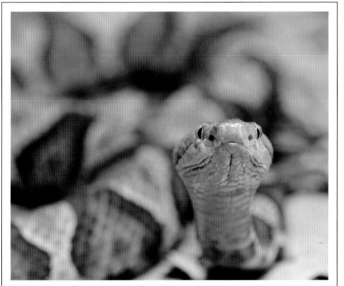

- Copperheads are the third of the three general types of North American pit vipers, and they, too, have no rattles.

- Their preferred habitat is deciduous forests and mixed woodlands, and they are found most often on rock outcroppings and ledges.

- Their habit of freezing when they feel threatened, instead of slithering hurriedly away, makes them the pit viper most likely to be stepped on.

- Treatment for bites of pit vipers is the same for all species.

Coral Snakes

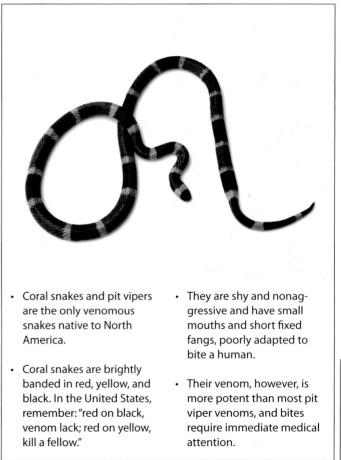

- Coral snakes and pit vipers are the only venomous snakes native to North America.

- Coral snakes are brightly banded in red, yellow, and black. In the United States, remember: "red on black, venom lack; red on yellow, kill a fellow."

- They are shy and nonaggressive and have small mouths and short fixed fangs, poorly adapted to bite a human.

- Their venom, however, is more potent than most pit viper venoms, and bites require immediate medical attention.

BITES & STINGS

SPIDERS

In the United States, three spiders are considered dangerous to humans

Spider bites fatal to humans are rare in the United States. The spiders considered dangerous are the black widow, recluse, and hobo.

Black widows seldom cause pain when they bite. There may be little or no redness and swelling at the site initially, but a small, red, slightly hard bump may form later. The bump may itch. Within ten to sixty minutes symptoms usually begin to occur. Pain and anxiety become intense. Severe muscular cramping often centers in the abdomen and back. Burning or numbness characteristically disturbs the patient's feet. Watch for headaches, nausea, vomiting, dizziness, heavy sweating—all common reactions.

Black Widows

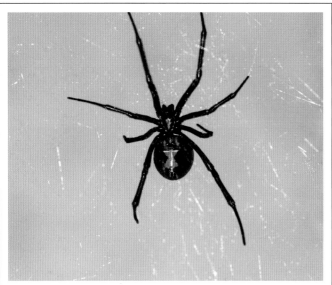

- Only the female black widow is dangerous, and she is the most dangerous spider in the United States.

- Typically, a red hourglass shape appears on the underside of her abdomen, but it is not always red and not always a complete hourglass.

- She builds a tattered web in which she waits for prey.

- Her venom usually causes severe cramping of abdominal and lower back muscles, and a doctor's care is required. Deaths in bitten humans are rare.

Recluse Spiders

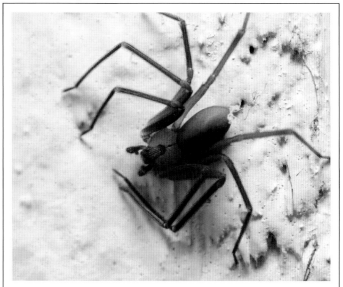

- Most recluse spiders have a violin or fiddle shape on the top of the front portion of their bodies, with the fiddle's head toward the rear of the spider.

- Unlike the widespread black widow, the recluse is predominately found in the midwestern states.

- Both sexes are equally venomous, and they are hunters, not web spinners.

- Bites are probably far less common than was once thought, but they leave a necrotic wound that requires a physician's care.

Within one to five hours of a recluse bite, a painful red blister appears where the fangs did their damage. Watch for the development of a bluish circle around the blister and a red, irritated circle beyond that—the characteristic "bull's-eye" lesion of the recluse. The patient may suffer chills, fever, a generalized weakness, and a diffuse rash. Sometimes the lesion resolves harmlessly over the next week or two. Sometimes it spreads irregularly as an enzyme in the spider's venom destroys the cells of the patient's skin and subcutaneous fat. This ulcerous tissue heals slowly and leaves a lasting scar.

Hobo Spiders

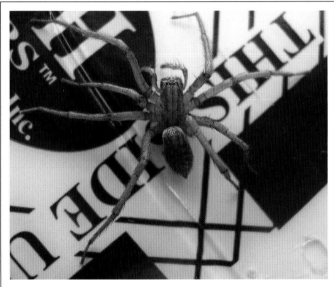

- Hobo spiders are nonnative, probably arriving from Europe on a ship about one hundred years ago. They are predominately residents of the northwestern states.

- They are similar to recluses in appearance, light brown in color with hairy legs, but lack the violin body shape.

- Hobo spider bites are rare, but they may leave a wound similar to that of a recluse bite and present similar signs and symptoms in the patient.

- First aid for spider bites includes applying cold and finding a doctor if the spider is venomous.

Avoiding Spider Bites

- Look into dark or hidden places before reaching in with hands or stepping in with bare feet.

- Regularly clean the hidden places in and under your house.

- Do not attempt to pick up or capture a spider.

BITES & STINGS

SCORPIONS

Serious harm from a scorpion sting in the United States is rare

Most victims of U.S. scorpion stings report no more pain than that inflicted by an irritated honeybee. An attack of the species *Centruroides* (Arizona bark scorpion) may be different. In North America only the *Centruroides* is a known killer of humans. Deaths, however, have almost exclusively been in small children, the elderly, and the severely allergic.

Arizona bark scorpions are usually the color of old straw—yellow or yellow with dark longitudinal stripes—and reach a length of 1–3 inches. Their pincers are long and slender as opposed to bulky and lobster-like. The sting, immediately and exquisitely painful, is increased by a light tap on the site. This scorpion is found only in Mexico and the extreme southwestern United States.

First aid for any scorpion sting should involve cooling the wound, which allows the patient's body to more easily break down the molecular structure of the venom. Cooling also

When a Scorpion Stings

- Relax.
- Put a cold pack on the sting site.
- Find a doctor for blurred vision, loss of bowel control, or jerky muscular spasms.

Scorpions

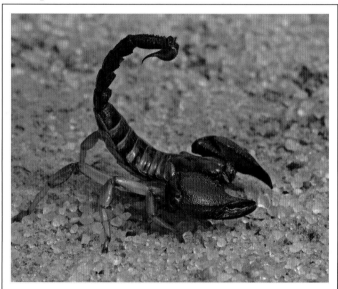

- All scorpions have eight legs and a pair of pincers for grasping their prey. And all scorpions are venomous.

- Almost all scorpions feed entirely on insects, but they sting humans when threatened.

- The "tail" is actually an extension of the abdomen with venom glands and a stinger at the hindmost end.

- The tail curls up over the scorpion's back to stab into the prey. Only rarely are stings from U.S. scorpions dangerous.

reduces pain. Use ice, chemical cold packs, or cool running water if available. On a warm night, a wet compress will help. Keep the patient calm and still. Panic and activity speed up the venom's spread.

If the scorpion was *Centruroides*, poststing manifestations may include heavy sweating, difficult swallowing, blurred vision, incontinence (loss of bowel control), jerky muscular reflexes, and respiratory distress.

······· RED ●LIGHT ·············

Find a doctor if the bitten person reports blurred vision, slurred speech, difficult swallowing, seizures, difficult breathing, or heart irregularities. Antivenins are available in many areas where dangerous scorpions live.

Centruroides

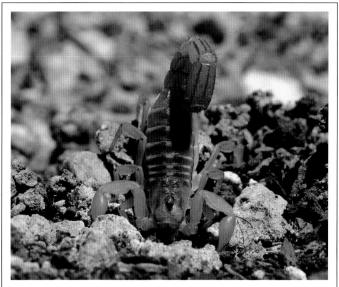

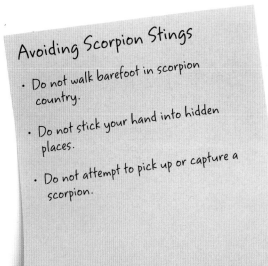

Avoiding Scorpion Stings

- Do not walk barefoot in scorpion country.

- Do not stick your hand into hidden places.

- Do not attempt to pick up or capture a scorpion.

- In the United States only the sting of *Centruroides exilicauda* has been documented to cause death in a human.

- They are a lean scorpion with slender pincers, seldom growing more than 3 inches in length. They are light brown.

- They are primarily inhabitants of the Sonoran Desert.

- Difficulty in breathing is a sign of serious envenomation, but there is no specific first-aid treatment. Hospitals in the area where these scorpions live have antivenom available.

BEES & WASPS

Bees and their relatives are the most dangerous U.S. animals

Bees, wasps (paper wasps, yellowjackets, hornets, for instance), and fire ants are related largely due to their habit of injecting venom when they sting. Most humans find the pain extremely annoying, and that's the end of the story. However, every year for an estimated fifty to one hundred people in the United States, the sting causes, usually in less than an hour, the end of life. Some experts guess the fatality rate runs even higher. Death almost always results from anaphylaxis, a severe allergic reaction (see "Severe Allergies").

Stings cause immediate pain, followed by redness and swelling, followed by itching. With any of these insects, ice packs generally ease the pain and swelling. Mild to moderate allergic reactions can be treated with an oral antihistamine. If severe difficulty in breathing results, only an injectable drug, epinephrine, available by prescription in preloaded syringes, reverses the reaction.

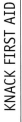

KNACK FIRST AID

Bees

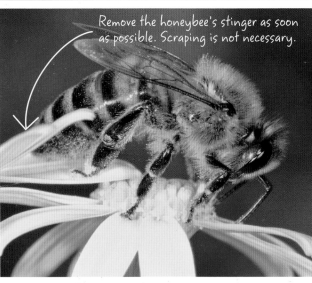

Remove the honeybee's stinger as soon as possible. Scraping is not necessary.

- Honeybees are not aggressive. They sting only when threatened, and their venom is weak, designed to discourage and not to kill.

- Their barbed stinger rips out of their bodies when they sting, and they die within twenty-four hours.

- The venom sac attached to each stinger will continue to pump out venom for up to twenty minutes. Remove the stinger as soon as possible by any means available.

- Killer bees are no more venomous than honeybees, but they attack in aggressive swarms.

Wasps

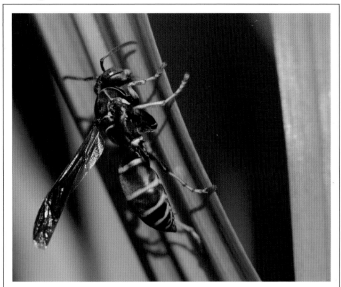

- The wasp family includes hornets and yellowjackets, and they sting more aggressively than bees, at least partially because they are protective of their nests.

- Their stingers are barbless, and one wasp can sting multiple times.

- Wasp venom is used for killing prey. It is more potent than bee venom, but it takes about one hundred simultaneous stings to threaten the life of an average human.

- Wasp stings should be washed to prevent infection, and cold packs will ease the pain.

If confronted by a bee or two or a wasp, stay calm and back away slowly. They don't like rapid movements, especially swatting movements. If attacked by a swarm, a rare occurrence, run for dense cover, lie face down, and cover your head with your hands.

Fire Ants

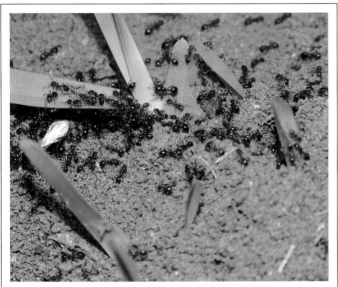

- Fire ants are relatives of bees and wasps due primarily to the fact that they sting with an apparatus at the tail end of their bodies.

- A fire ant will grab hold with mandibles and deliver multiple stings before letting go.

- Fire ants are notoriously aggressive, attacking anything that disturbs the mounds in which they live.

- As with bees and wasps, death by fire ant sting, though not common, is possible from an anaphylactic reaction.

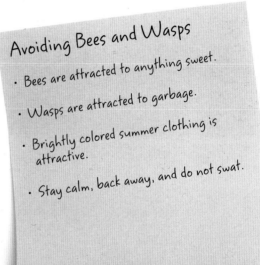

Avoiding Bees and Wasps

- Bees are attracted to anything sweet.

- Wasps are attracted to garbage.

- Brightly colored summer clothing is attractive.

- Stay calm, back away, and do not swat.

BITES & STINGS

GENDER-SPECIFIC OVERVIEW

Injuries and illnesses involving the genitalia are embarrassing as well as frightening

Injuries involving the genitalia can be embarrassing, frightening, and, from time to time, life-threatening. A variety of illnesses can also affect the reproductive systems of males and females, and they, too, can be serious. A first-aid provider might have to deal with some of these problems.

Both you and the patient will appreciate a private place to talk. The patient will benefit if you can maintain eye contact while being straightforward, respectful, and nonjudgmental. Use proper medical terminology and/or terms that you both understand, and avoid jokes or slang that risk making you both uncomfortable. The patient needs to provide accurate information, as always, but in this case a member

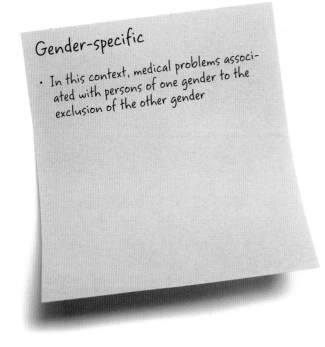

Gender-specific

- In this context, medical problems associated with persons of one gender to the exclusion of the other gender

Privacy

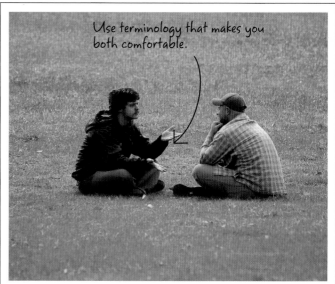

Use terminology that makes you both comfortable.

- Gender-specific medical problems are often a source of embarrassment to the patient.

- It is almost always easier for the patient to discuss such problems with someone of the same gender, even if that person is not the most trained first-aid provider.

- Find a private place to talk out of hearing of other people.

- Discuss the problem openly and directly. Do nothing by word choice, tone of voice, or body language that increases the emotional discomfort of the patient.

of the patient's sex is often better able to put the patient at ease. A member of the patient's sex should be present before and during any physical exam—especially where minors are involved—unless it is impossible. You may choose to explain to a competent companion with less medical training, someone of the same sex, what you require in a physical examination and ask that person to perform the exam.

Inspection

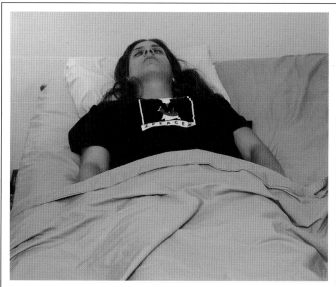

More Tips

- Use appropriate names for anatomical parts.
- Make eye contact as much as possible.
- Be respectful.
- Be nonjudgmental.

- If physical inspection of the genitalia is required, it is critical, in almost all cases, to have someone of the same gender perform the inspection.

- This may require having an untrained person perform the inspection, reporting what he or she observes to you in as much detail as possible.

- Expose no more of the patient than is absolutely necessary.

- Take no more time than is absolutely necessary to perform the inspection.

CRAMPS

Several problems, some serious and some not, are associated with the menstrual cycle

Abdominal cramping in women is most often associated with their menstrual cycle. An awareness of the patient's normal cycle is important in making an assessment. Abnormal cramping will be cause for concern.

Dysmenorrhea is pain in association with menstruation. Possible causes include prostaglandins, which cause the uterus

to cramp; endometritis, which is inflammation of the endometrium; pelvic inflammatory disease; or anatomic anomalies such as a displaced uterus. If a woman is unsure of the cause of her cramps, she should be evaluated by a physician.

Some women describe cramps in the lower abdomen on the right or left side or in the back during the middle of the

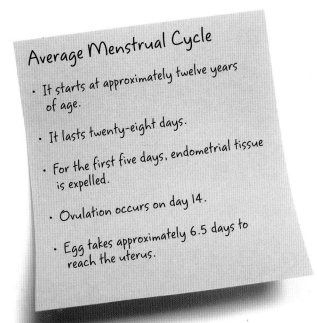

Average Menstrual Cycle

- It starts at approximately twelve years of age.

- It lasts twenty-eight days.

- For the first five days, endometrial tissue is expelled.

- Ovulation occurs on day 14.

- Egg takes approximately 6.5 days to reach the uterus.

Pain

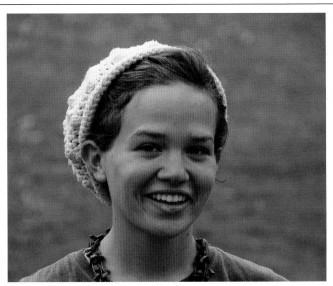

- Cramping is often associated with menstruation.

- Cramping may occur in the lower abdomen on the right or left side or in the back in the middle of the menstrual cycle when the ovary releases an egg, and the pain may be sudden, sharp, and severe.

- Over-the-counter pain medications and general support may be all you can offer.

- Some women report benefits from heat packs, massages to the lower back, and/or relaxation exercises.

menstrual cycle. This is when the ovary releases an egg. The pain is sometimes accompanied by bloody vaginal discharge. This is called "*mittelschmerz*" from the German *mittel* for "middle" and *schmerz* for "pain." The pain may be sudden, sharp, and severe enough to be confused with appendicitis or ectopic pregnancy (see "Ectopic Pregnancy & Miscarriage"). Ask the patient if she is menstruating. Has she ever had this pain before? Typically, a woman will have had similar cramping in the past. Any light bleeding or pain should cease within thirty-six hours.

Drugs such as ibuprofen usually reduce the pain. Doing relaxation exercises such as yoga and massaging the lower back or abdomen may help reduce pain. Applying heat to the abdomen or lower back may also help reduce pain. A change in diet may help. Decreasing the amount of salt, caffeine, and alcohol in the diet while increasing the B vitamins—especially B6, found in brewer's yeast, peanuts, rice, sunflower seeds, and whole grains—can offer some relief during the acute phase of the cramps. Because exercise causes endorphins (natural opiates) to be released by the brain, many women find that cramps diminish when they participate in strenuous exercise.

Cramps and Pregnancy

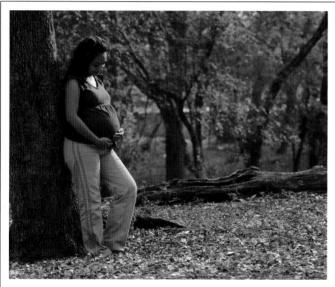

- Abdominal cramping is not generally associated with pregnancy until the onset of contractions prior to delivery.

- If a woman is experiencing cramping earlier in pregnancy, it could be a signal of a serious problem.

- Cramping could signal an impending miscarriage that will be fatal to the fetus but rarely a serious medical problem for the woman.

- Cramping early in pregnancy could signal an ectopic pregnancy that requires immediate transport to a hospital.

Serious Cramping

- Associated with unusual and/or unusually heavy vaginal bleeding

- Associated with vaginal bleeding and the possibility of pregnancy

- Associated with a high fever

YEAST & OTHER INFECTIONS
Women are susceptible to several infections that men are not

There are three major types of vaginal infections: *yeast* (fungus), *bacterial vaginosis* (bacteria), and *Trichomonas* (a parasitic protozoan). For the purposes of assessment, the symptoms are similar, and initial treatment is the same.

Signals of infection include redness, soreness, or itching in the vaginal area. There may be an excessive or malodorous discharge from the vagina. There may also be a burning sensation during urination.

Women with a history of vaginal yeast infections have often already chosen their preferred treatment. There are common medications available over the counter and used to treat yeast infections. (Women with bacterial vaginosis or Trichomonas will require antibiotic treatment.) Acetaminophen and warm, moist compresses should provide symptomatic relief from the pain. Itching often responds to cool compresses and over-the-counter 0.5 percent hydrocortisone cream. If these

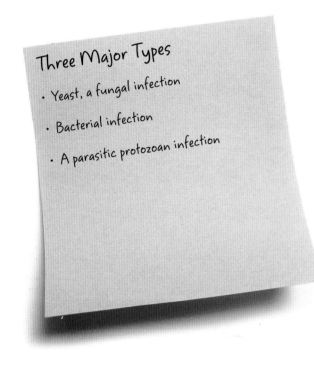

Three Major Types

- Yeast, a fungal infection

- Bacterial infection

- A parasitic protozoan infection

Treatment

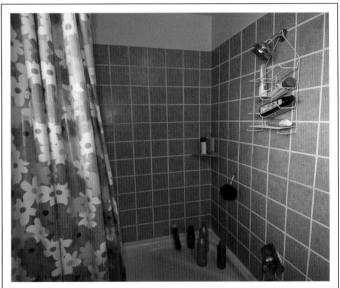

- The perineal area (the vaginal and rectal areas) should be cleaned with warm water and soap and kept clean.

- Acetaminophen (following the directions on the label) and warm, moist compresses should provide some relief for the pain.

- Itching, which can be severe, often responds to cool compresses and over-the-counter 0.5 percent hydrocortisone cream.

- Coffee, alcohol, and sugar-rich foods—all of which alter the pH of the vagina—should be avoided.

treatments don't provide relief within forty-eight hours, the patient should be evaluated by a physician. An untreated infection can develop into pelvic inflammatory disease.

To help prevent vaginal infections, women should take care to clean the perineal area with plain water or a mild soap daily and to wear cotton underpants and loose outer pants. Unlike cotton, nylon doesn't allow air to circulate, thus giving bacteria a moist place to grow. Women should avoid coffee, alcohol, and sugar when the signs and symptoms of infection exist.

Specific Medications

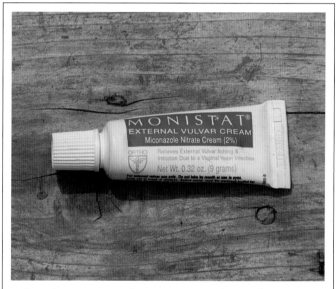

- Over-the-counter medications include several topical agents that fight yeast infections. Women who suffer infections often are encouraged to try several to find the one that works best for them.

- A prescription-only oral medication, fluconazole, cures almost all yeast infections.

- Infections that do not respond to home treatment are likely to be bacterial or protozoan, and these two types of infections require antibiotic therapy.

· · · · · · · · · · · · · · · RED ● LIGHT · · · · · · · · · · · · · ·

If the patient does not respond to treatment at home and find relief within forty-eight hours, she should be evaluated by a physician. The condition may be a more serious infection.

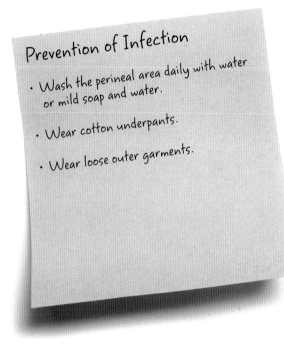

Prevention of Infection

- Wash the perineal area daily with water or mild soap and water.

- Wear cotton underpants.

- Wear loose outer garments.

185

URINARY TRACT INFECTIONS

Both females and males are susceptible to infections of the urinary tract

Urinary tract infections (UTIs) are relatively rare in men but common in women due to the relatively short length of the urethra through which pathogens are introduced, causing the problem. Untreated, the infection can affect the urethra, bladder, ureters, even the kidneys.

Urinary tract infections cause increased frequency or urgency of urination with decreased urine output and/or a burning sensation during urination. The patient usually complains of pain above the pubic bone and a heavy urine odor with the morning urination. Blood and/or pus may be present in the urine. Urinary tract infections can progress to kidney infections. If the kidneys are infected, the patient usually

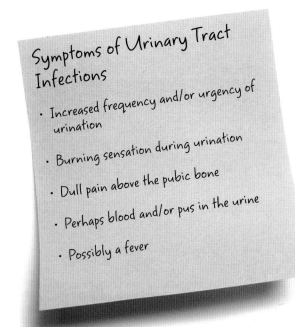

Symptoms of Urinary Tract Infections

- Increased frequency and/or urgency of urination
- Burning sensation during urination
- Dull pain above the pubic bone
- Perhaps blood and/or pus in the urine
- Possibly a fever

Drinking Water

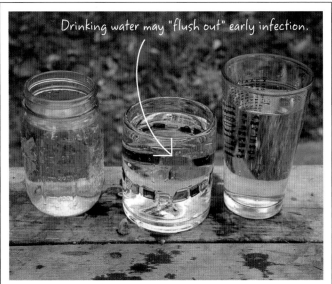

Drinking water may "flush out" early infection.

- If a urinary tract infection is caught early, the patient should be encouraged to drink as much water as possible. Drinking will be an act of discipline and not based on thirst.

- Repeated emptying of the bladder often flushes out the germs causing the infection.

- During treatment, the patient needs to get as much rest as possible.

- The perineal area should be cleaned daily with water or mild soap and water.

complains of pain in the small of the back where the ribs join the backbone and usually complains of tenderness when that area is palpated. The patient may have a fever.

UTIs may be treated early and successfully by having the patient drink as much water as possible. Repeated emptying of the bladder may "flush out" the offending pathogens. A patient with a UTI should get as much rest as possible. The perineal area should be cleaned with water and mild soap daily.

Medications

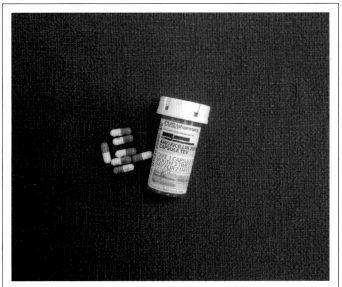

- Infections that are not caught early enough or that do not for other reasons respond to superhydration need to be treated with an antibiotic.

- A physician should be consulted for the specific antibiotic and the prescription.

- As always, antibiotics need to be taken for the full length of the prescription, even if the patient feels well before completion.

- Additionally, an over-the-counter medication, phenazopyridine, often relieves the pain experienced on urination.

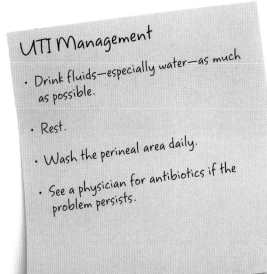

UTI Management
- Drink fluids—especially water—as much as possible.
- Rest.
- Wash the perineal area daily.
- See a physician for antibiotics if the problem persists.

EPIDIDYMITIS

This inflammation of the male genitalia tends to come on slowly, perhaps over days

The epididymis is a structure in the scrotum. There are two, attached to the back of each testis, and they store spermatozoa until maturity. *Epididymitis* is an inflammation of an epididymis, a problem caused most often by bacteria that invade via the urinary tract, and sometimes caused by nonbacterial agents. It is the most common cause of

scrotal pain and inflammation, and it can lead to loss of a testicle. Epididymitis is not caused by traumatic injury to the scrotum.

The patient suffers from pain in the scrotum that can range from mild to severe. The pain will possibly be accompanied by fever. The scrotum is often unusually warm and red and

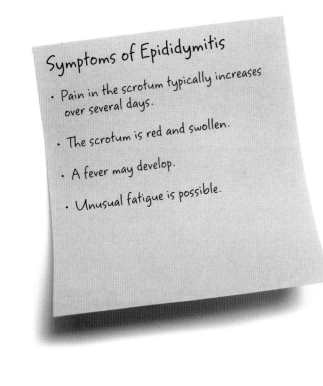

Symptoms of Epididymitis
- Pain in the scrotum typically increases over several days.
- The scrotum is red and swollen.
- A fever may develop.
- Unusual fatigue is possible.

Treatment 1

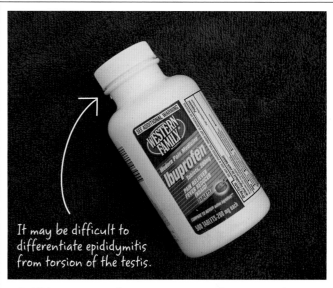

It may be difficult to differentiate epididymitis from torsion of the testis.

- Epididymitis is an inflammation that may be caused by a sexually transmitted disease (STD) germ such as chlamydia, gonorrhea, or syphilis, or another non-STD bacteria. It is not the result of trauma to the testicles.

- You can help relieve the pain with a nonsteroidal anti-inflammatory drug such as aspirin, ibuprofen, or naproxen. If a fever develops, these same drugs, along with adequate hydration, will benefit the patient.

- Antibiotics, however, are most often required for resolution of the disease.

swollen. Epididymitis tends to come on slowly, perhaps over several days, unlike torsion of the testis, which sometimes comes on rapidly (see "Torsion of the Testis"). The pain of epididymitis, however, may be reported by the patient as "sudden."

The immediate treatment is bed rest and support of the scrotum with a jock strap or whatever can be improvised to create support for the testicles. A dose of a nonsteroidal anti-inflammatory drug (NSAID) such as aspirin or ibuprofen may decrease the fever and pain.

Treatment 2

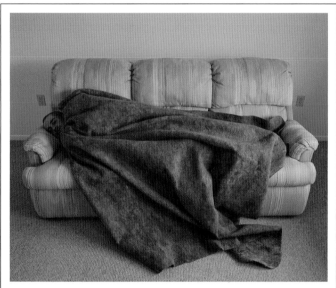

- Bed rest is required for this patient.

- Most patients will also further benefit from support of the scrotum, ideally provided by a jock strap.

- Cold compresses are sometimes useful in reducing pain.

- With antibiotic therapy, recovery is almost always complete, and loss of a testicle is rare. In severe cases, however, the patient may be admitted to the hospital for several days. If the problem has an STD as the cause, the sexual partner will need treatment as well.

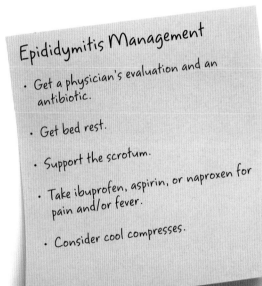

Epididymitis Management

- Get a physician's evaluation and an antibiotic.

- Get bed rest.

- Support the scrotum.

- Take ibuprofen, aspirin, or naproxen for pain and/or fever.

- Consider cool compresses.

TORSION OF THE TESTIS
Causes can be dramatically violent or deceptively nonviolent, but treatment is the same

Torsion of the testis is a twisting of the testis within the scrotum. Mechanisms for testicular torsion could be as dramatic as engaging in violent physical activity or as simple as rolling over in bed. The ductus deferens and its accompanying blood vessels become twisted, decreasing the blood supply to the testis. If the blood supply is totally cut off, the testis dies.

With many patients, the scrotum is suddenly and intensely full of pain, sometimes rendering the patient unable to move. The scrotum grows red and swollen, and the testis may appear slightly elevated on the affected side. The pain, however, can come on slowly, and the other "classic" signs and symptoms may be absent.

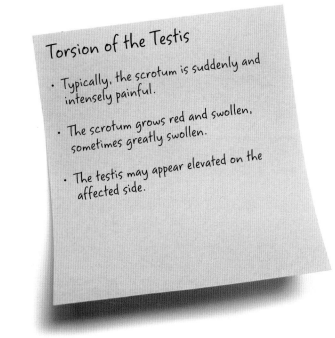

Torsion of the Testis

- Typically, the scrotum is suddenly and intensely painful.

- The scrotum grows red and swollen, sometimes greatly swollen.

- The testis may appear elevated on the affected side.

Treatment 1

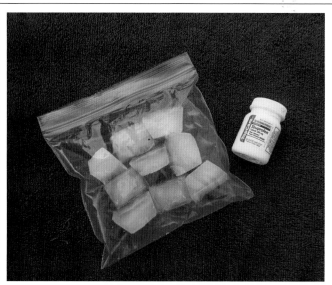

- The patient needs to have the testicle twisted back into the proper alignment.

- Some patients suffer torsion of the testis relatively often, and they are often able to rotate their own testicle back into its proper position.

- Until rotation is accomplished, the patient may benefit from the application of cold to the scrotum with either an ice pack or a cool compress.

- Some pain relief is possible with an over-the-counter medication such as ibuprofen.

Cool compresses and pain medication will provide some relief. A jock strap will elevate the scrotum and may increase blood flow to the testis. The patient, ideally, should be transported for treatment immediately. If transport will be delayed, you may attempt to rotate the affected testicle back into position. Because most testicles rotate "inward," a gentle lifting and a gentle rotation "outward" may give immediate relief. If that doesn't work, perhaps the testicle rotated in the opposite direction, so rotate the testicle two turns in the opposite direction. No more than two attempts are recommended.

Treatment 2

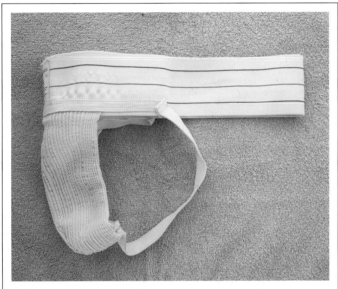

- Some patients with testicular torsion find that they are unable to walk. If help is on the way, remaining on their back may relieve some pain for these patients.

- The use of a jock strap that elevates the scrotum may increase the blood supply to the testicle and/or improve mobility.

- Without a jock strap, you may be able to improvise a sling that lifts the scrotum.

- A relatively simple surgery can prevent the reoccurrence of torsion of the testis.

RED ● LIGHT

If the victim of torsion of the testis does not have the twist of the testis removed within twenty-four hours, the testicle may be lost.

Testicular Torsion Management
- Call 911 immediately.
- Keep the patient at rest on his back.
- If walking is required, apply a jock strap.
- Cold packs and ibuprofen may be beneficial if transport is delayed.

191

ECTOPIC PREGNANCY & MISCARRIAGE

Quick recognition and transportation of a pregnant woman may be all that can save her life

When the developing embryo implants in a fallopian tube (or, rarely, in another pelvic site) instead of inside the uterus, the woman has an *ectopic* pregnancy. The embryo invades the wall of the tube, and blood vessels in the tube enlarge dramatically. Eventually, the blood vessels will rupture, and the woman will bleed into her abdominal cavity. The bleeding

can be fierce, and, in all cases, death is imminent without emergency surgery to repair the damage. Shortly after the first signs of pregnancy appear, the woman may notice mild cramping and vaginal bleeding. Pain and vaginal bleeding increase as the placenta increasingly invades the tube. The woman needs a medical facility immediately.

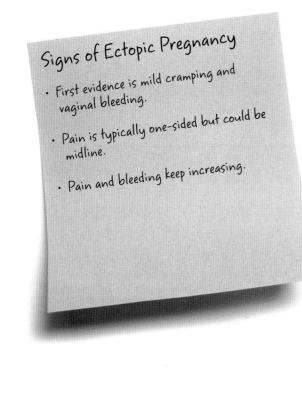

Signs of Ectopic Pregnancy

- First evidence is mild cramping and vaginal bleeding.

- Pain is typically one-sided but could be midline.

- Pain and bleeding keep increasing.

Ectopic Pregnancy Treatment

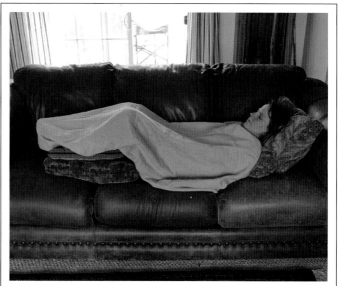

- With an ectopic pregnancy, the placenta is literally eating its way into the wall of the fallopian tube.

- Eventually large blood vessels will rupture, and internal bleeding will be intense and rapidly life-threatening.

- The patient should be treated for shock: kept still and lying down, covered, and offered reassurance.

- But only rapid transport to a hospital saves the patient once large vessels rupture. Nothing can be done in the field.

A *miscarriage*, or *spontaneous abortion*, occurs commonly in the first few weeks of pregnancy. Some women have a miscarriage before they know they are pregnant. Women who miscarry later in pregnancy usually experience menstrual-like cramps that increase in severity and frequency. Vaginal bleeding begins. After one or two hours of painful cramps and unusual bleeding, the woman typically passes fetal tissue and the placenta. Most miscarriages do not threaten the woman physically, but physicians can deliver drugs to ease the pain. Occasionally the woman needs definitive aid to stop the bleeding.

•••••••••••••• RED ● LIGHT ••••••••••••••

If there is any chance that cramps and bleeding could be indicating a patient with an ectopic pregnancy, the woman must be transported to a hospital as rapidly as possible.

Miscarriage

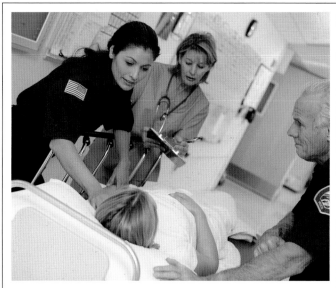

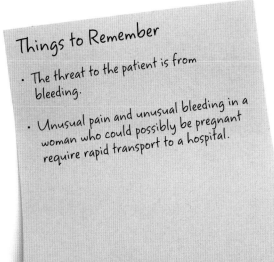

Things to Remember

- The threat to the patient is from bleeding.

- Unusual pain and unusual bleeding in a woman who could possibly be pregnant require rapid transport to a hospital.

- A miscarriage often occurs early in pregnancy, sometimes even before a woman knows she is pregnant.

- In an early miscarriage, the woman may have a slightly delayed and heavy period as the only evidence of her miscarriage.

- A miscarriage is a natural process that can usually take place without medical intervention, even when the pregnancy is advanced.

- Physicians can often provide drugs that shorten the process and ease the amount of discomfort involved.

PLACENTA PREVIA & ABRUPTION

Emergencies associated with the placenta must be recognized and managed quickly

Vaginal bleeding during the last three months of pregnancy may signal a serious problem with the placenta. And two problems can be life-threatening to mother and baby.

When the placenta implants right over the cervix, it may separate from the uterus when the cervix begins to thin and dilate prior to labor. This condition is known as *placenta previa*. The

bleeding from the vagina can be painless, but it is most often life-threateningly profuse. Only a cesarean section (C-section), surgically delivering the baby, saves mother and baby.

Fortunately, due to ultrasound, most women know if their placentas are implanted dangerously and make plans ahead of time to deal with it.

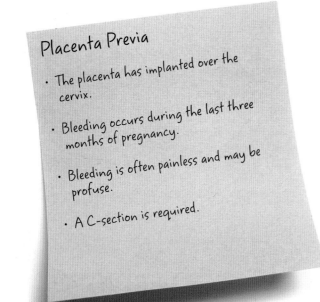

Placenta Previa

- The placenta has implanted over the cervix.

- Bleeding occurs during the last three months of pregnancy.

- Bleeding is often painless and may be profuse.

- A C-section is required.

Placenta Previa

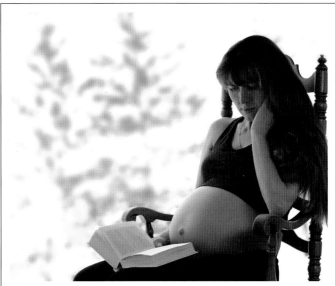

- There is very little that can be done for this woman outside a hospital.

- Fortunately, most women today know well in advance if they have placenta previa due to the regular use of ultrasounds.

- The woman should not plan extended trips, especially trips that take her far from a hospital, during the last three months of pregnancy.

- The woman should limit her physical activity significantly during the last two months of pregnancy.

The second problem, *placental abruption*, occurs when the placenta separates, either partially or completely, from the wall of the uterus well ahead of the woman's delivery date. When the placenta separates, painful contractions begin and increase in frequency and severity. The pain can become very severe. The separation usually causes vaginal bleeding that can range from mild to severe.

Partial separations can sometimes be managed without surgery. Complete separations require immediate surgery and usually result in loss of the baby.

Placental Abruption

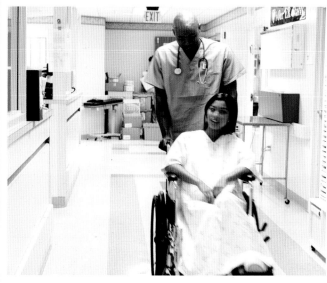

- A placental abruption can be partial or complete, depending on how much of the placenta separates from the uterine wall.

- Partial abruptions can sometimes be treated without surgery, once again depending on the extent of the separation.

- A complete abruption is completely catastrophic for the baby and potentially fatal to the mother.

- Abruptions are more common when the woman has high blood pressure, and they can be caused by trauma or cocaine use.

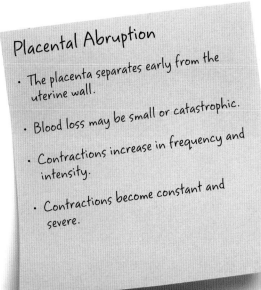

Placental Abruption

- The placenta separates early from the uterine wall.

- Blood loss may be small or catastrophic.

- Contractions increase in frequency and intensity.

- Contractions become constant and severe.

195

EMERGENCY DELIVERY 1
If the baby will be delivered outside a hospital, you must be prepared

How do you know if you have time to reach the hospital when a woman goes into labor? Or will you have to prepare to help with the delivery then and there?

Almost all first pregnancies involve at least four to six hours of hard labor. In a fifth pregnancy, on the other hand, labor may last less than one hour. If the delivery is premature, it usually happens more quickly. Labor at six weeks before the due date can be several hours shorter. If the woman has had a "gush" of clear fluid, her membranes have ruptured, and you can expect the baby 25 percent sooner than if her membranes are intact. With contractions coming every two to three minutes and lasting about forty-five seconds each,

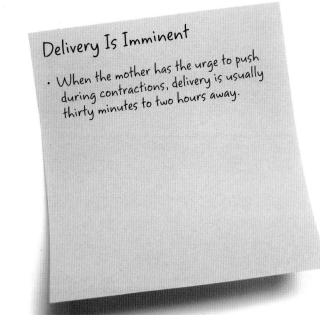

Delivery Is Imminent

- When the mother has the urge to push during contractions, delivery is usually thirty minutes to two hours away.

Position of the Mother

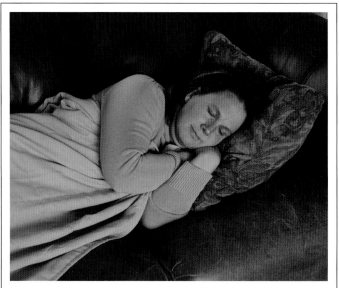

- When you have decided you do not have time to reach a hospital before delivery, devote your attention to the delivery.

- Remove the patient's clothing, position her on her left side, and keep her covered to prevent body heat loss.

- The left side position maximizes healthy blood flow to the patient and to the baby.

- The left side position provides room between the baby's head and the bed, which will be covered in fluids lost by the mother during delivery.

you can expect the baby within one or two hours. When the woman says she needs to push, birth is imminent.

Outside a hospital, the best position for the mother who is going to deliver is on her left side. It is usually best for her to deliver in this position as well. Garments must be removed—you will be placing the newborn on Mom's bare chest—and access to the baby must be as easy as possible. But keep the mother covered with soft, clean material to prevent heat loss.

ZOOM

Prior to delivery, with warm water and soap wash your hands, the mother's hands, and her vaginal and anal area, and then rinse thoroughly with clean, warm water.

Washing

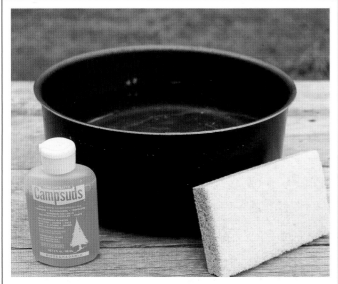

- You need to wash your hands well with soap and warm water and dry your hands with a clean cloth or towel.

- You don't need to boil water, but you do need a couple of pots of warm water, soap, and a clean cloth.

- You need to wash the mother's hands and her perineal area (her vaginal and rectal areas).

- You need to rinse the perineal area well with clean water.

Delivery Is Really Imminent

- When the top of the baby's head, the crown, appears during contractions, delivery is not far away.

197

EMERGENCY DELIVERY 2
With most births, the steps to take during delivery do not vary

Delivery of the infant should be slow and not explosive to prevent damage to the baby.

The baby's head descends a little with each contraction. When the baby's head down to the ears is visible outside the vagina, the rest of the baby will come more easily because the baby gets smaller below the ears. At this point the mother will also have the most urgent need to push the baby out as quickly as possible. Place your hand on the top of the baby's head to *gently* slow delivery of the head. Tell Mom to stop pushing. You may have to speak very loudly. Then ask her to bear down gently. You want the head to come out at the same speed it has been descending up to that point.

When the head is fully out, ask Mom to stop pushing again. The head is usually face down, rarely face up. Baby's head will rotate to one side or the other. You can assist by very *gently* rotating the head to the side. It will rotate to one side

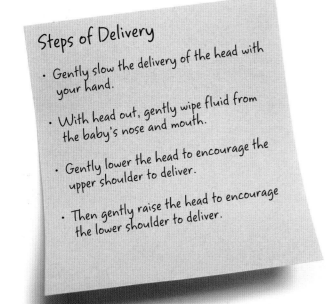

Steps of Delivery

- Gently slow the delivery of the head with your hand.

- With head out, gently wipe fluid from the baby's nose and mouth.

- Gently lower the head to encourage the upper shoulder to deliver.

- Then gently raise the head to encourage the lower shoulder to deliver.

Newborn

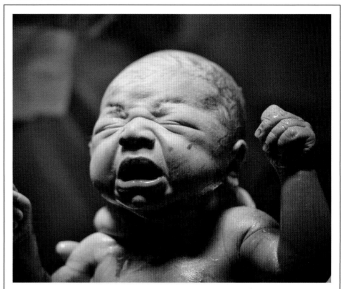

- Remember: The little body will be slippery!

- Keep the baby's head slightly lower than the body, and keep the head and body turned to the side to allow fluids to drain from the baby's airway.

- Wipe the baby's skin dry with the cleanest, softest material available. Be vigorous. This will also stimulate the baby to breathe.

- Rubbing the back is an especially effective way to stimulate breathing. Baby can rest on Mother's bare chest and abdomen while you do this.

very easily. Now gently wipe the fluid from Baby's nose and mouth.

With the next contraction, Mom can finish pushing out the baby. If you lower Baby's head slightly, it will encourage the upper shoulder to deliver. Then you can slightly lift Baby's head to help the lower shoulder out. Remind Mom to keep pushing under control to keep the delivery slow and smooth.

With Baby out, make sure that your grasp is secure, and, supporting the head, hold him or her with the head slightly

lower than the rest of the body to allow fluids to leak out of the nose and mouth. Place Baby on Mom's bare chest in a position that keeps the head lower than the rest of the little body.

Cutting the Cord

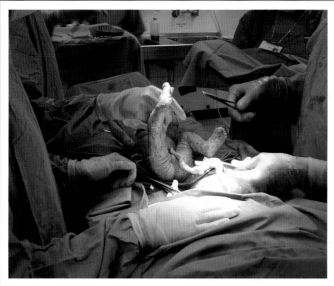

- Keep the baby covered and on the mother's bare skin. Preventing heat loss from the baby is critical!

- Carefully and tightly tie the umbilical cord with two pieces of wide string, such as clean shoelaces, several inches from the baby and about 1 inch apart.

- Cut the cord between the strings.

- If any blood leaks from the baby's side of the cord, pinch it off immediately. Baby has little blood to lose.

The Placenta

- The placenta will deliver in five to ten minutes.

- Apply gentle, slow traction to the cord to encourage delivery.

- It is best to grasp and continuously twist the placenta as it delivers.

- With the placenta out, immediately massage the mother's uterus.

- Keep massaging for at least ten minutes.

COMPLICATIONS OF DELIVERY

The baby can assume numerous complicated positions during delivery

Several complications are associated with the position of the baby in the birth canal. Some you may be able to handle—and some not.

If you see the umbilical cord wrapped around the baby's neck, attempt to slip the cord gently over the head. Usually, the cord is loose enough to slip over easily. If the cord is too tight to move, you need to tie two pieces of string around the cord tightly, about 1 inch apart, and cut the cord. Delivery must not be delayed after the cutting.

If you see part of the umbilical cord presenting first in the vagina, it is called a *prolapsed cord*. During delivery, pressure on a prolapsed cord often cuts off the vital blood supply to

KNACK FIRST AID

Breech Presentation

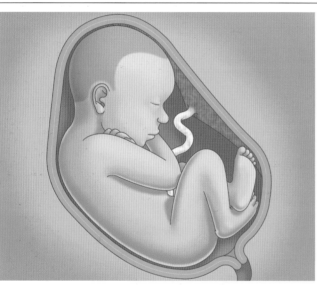

- Baby's feet or buttocks are coming out first.

- Rapidly transport the mother to a hospital.

- If transport is delayed, you can do nothing until Baby is delivered most of the way.

- Then gently reach into the vagina, place a finger in the baby's mouth, keep the chin down to the baby's chest, and hope for delivery.

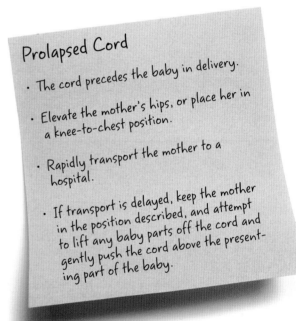

Prolapsed Cord

- The cord precedes the baby in delivery.

- Elevate the mother's hips, or place her in a knee-to-chest position.

- Rapidly transport the mother to a hospital.

- If transport is delayed, keep the mother in the position described, and attempt to lift any baby parts off the cord and gently push the cord above the presenting part of the baby.

the baby. Tell Mom to stop pushing, and elevate her hips. You may be able to lift the presenting part of the baby off the life-sustaining cord, but most often only rapid transport to a medical facility saves Mom and/or Baby.

If you see Baby's buttocks or feet first, you are looking at a *breech presentation*. Tell the mother to stop pushing. Although breech presentations can be successfully delivered, the process is complicated, most often requiring the skill of a professional. Rapid transport is critical.

················· GREEN ● LIGHT ··············

Fortunately, more than 98 percent of babies are born head first, the position of the baby that creates the fewest possible complications during delivery.

Umbilical Cord around Neck

- With Baby's head out, you see the umbilical cord.

- It is almost always loose.

- Slip it up and over the baby's head.

- Continue the delivery.

Avoiding Complications

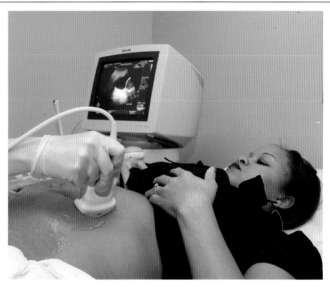

- Regular prenatal check-ups with ultrasounds reveal many complications.

- Mother should not travel far from home during the final month.

- Complications are almost always dealt with better in hospitals.

MOTHER & NEWBORN CARE

Delivery is not over until the mother and newborn are properly cared for

For the best outcome, proper care of the newborn is extremely important. At most births, drying and stimulating the baby need to occur prior to cutting the cord (see "Emergency Delivery 2").

With the baby on the bare skin of the mother's chest or upper abdomen, wipe Baby dry with the cleanest, softest material available. Pay particular attention to the hair and scalp. Drying prevents body heat loss, a critical factor with newborns. Be vigorous with your drying. Rubbing Baby's back is an especially safe and effective way to stimulate breathing. Baby will start to wake up and fuss. Fussing and crying provide adequate oxygen to Baby, and that wakes

Newborn Care

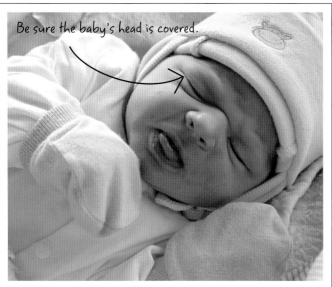

Be sure the baby's head is covered.

- Newborns have a critical and immediate need for two things: a clear airway and warmth. Everything else can wait.

- As mentioned earlier, after airway clearing, the baby needs to be thoroughly dried with the softest, cleanest material available.

- Pay particular attention to the hair and scalp.

- Baby should then be wrapped in clean, dry, soft material or dressed in clean, dry, soft clothing.

- Be sure to provide a covering for the baby's head.

Mother Care

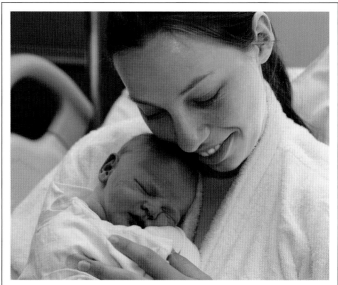

- Most of the immediate care that the new mother needs will be met when she holds her baby.

- After the initial massage of her uterus for at least ten minutes, repeat uterine massage if vaginal bleeding continues or reoccurs.

- The mother will likely be dehydrated, so keep plenty of liquids handy for drinking. Encourage the mother to drink because she might not think of it.

- Keep the mother covered to prevent loss of her body heat.

Baby up more, and the cycle continues. When you finish the drying process, feel the umbilical cord. You should easily find the baby's pulse in the cord. Baby's heart should be beating approximately 140 times per minute. If the heart is beating less than one hundred times per minute, an unusual occurrence, perform mouth-to-nose-and-mouth rescue breathing until Baby responds (see "Infant CPR").

Wrap Baby warmly in soft, dry material, including covering for the head, and give the baby to the mother.

Nursing

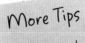

- Baby does not need any liquids at all for twenty-four hours, even though newborns may try to nurse for the first hour or so after birth.

- The act of nursing causes the release of pitocin from the mother's pituitary gland.

- Pitocin is a hormone necessary for the milk let-down reflex, and it also causes uterine contractions that help slow postpartum bleeding from the mother.

- Nursing also helps start the mother-child bonding process.

More Tips

- Baby can be kept adequately warm by being held against Mother's bare skin and covered with insulating material.

- Mother will be exhausted and should be encouraged to rest.

- Both mother and child should be evaluated by a physician, but speed is not required if both are doing well.

INJURIES TO CHILDREN
Treatment of injuries to children is not always the same as treatment of injuries to adults

Young children are often unable to tell you what hurts, making assessment a challenge. Older children may respond to injuries with a lot of drama, making it difficult to evaluate their level of pain. Some general guidelines will be helpful.

Expect to spend more time with a child than with an adult patient. You may have to spend time establishing trust, even if you are a parent of the child. Stay calm. Do not rush. Try giving a small child a favorite toy as a distraction. And avoid saying, "This won't hurt," because it might.

Children can go into shock (see "Shock") faster than adults, but they give clues to shock differently. Check for a rapid heart rate, yes, but look for apathy, mottled skin, and a warm

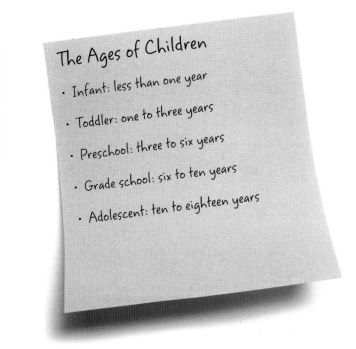

The Ages of Children

- Infant: less than one year
- Toddler: one to three years
- Preschool: three to six years
- Grade school: six to ten years
- Adolescent: ten to eighteen years

Musculoskeletal Injuries

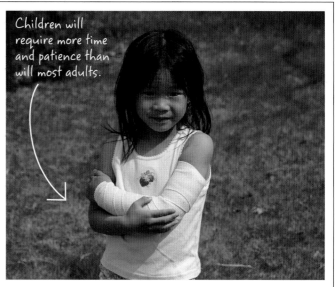

Children will require more time and patience than will most adults.

- Watch for aggressive guarding (overprotection of the injury site by the child) as a sign of significant injury.

- Any significant tenderness near a joint, especially near an ankle, knee, or elbow, should be considered a growth plate injury and evaluated as soon as pos-

sible by a physician.

- Children are susceptible to "greenstick" fractures in which the young, soft bone bends and partially breaks. The arm or leg obviously bends abnormally at the fracture site. Splint children as you do adults.

body with cold arms and legs as indicators.

Injuries that cause significant tenderness near a joint (see "Check Joints & Bones") have to be considered a growth plate injury and evaluated by a physician to ensure proper bone development. There are, however, no special considerations involved in splinting a child's bone or joint injury. Minor strains and sprains are treated the same as an adult's.

Wound Management

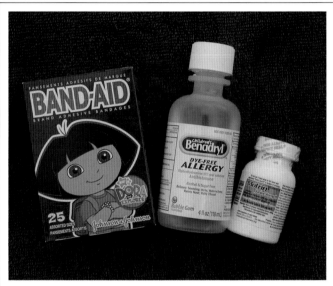

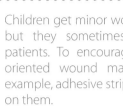

- Small bodies contain less blood, and serious bleeding in children requires your utmost speed in applying and maintaining direct pressure on the wound.

- Antiseptic towelettes that contain benzalkonium chloride do not sting and make excellent cleaning swabs for small wounds. They can also be used to clean unbroken skin.

- Bright materials, like those with cartoon characters on them, distract children from their wounds. Keep an eye on bandaged wounds because children tend to remove bandages often.

Approaching the Pediatric Patient

- Stay calm, or at least act calm.

- Expect to take more time, especially to build trust.

- Distract the child with toys or games.

- Examine uninjured body parts before the injured part.

- Do not focus on the injury and ignore the child.

HEAT, COLD, & CHILDREN
Kids gain and lose body heat from the environment faster than do adults

Little bodies gain and lose core heat faster than do big bodies. The younger the child, the less developed the internal heat regulating system and the larger the surface area in relation to the body mass.

Allow your children time to acclimatize to heat. It will take them longer than it will take you. Early in the hot season or early into a trip to an area hotter than your child is used to, go easy for the first few days, and increase the activity level progressively. The human body becomes increasingly able to withstand the heat.

In cold weather, you must be responsible for dressing your children appropriately. They may—or, more often, may

Heat

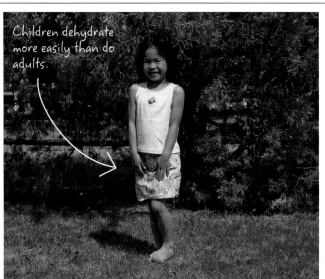

Children dehydrate more easily than do adults.

- Overheated children appear flushed, have a rapid heartbeat, may seem mildly confused, may complain of a headache and nausea, and seem weak.

- Move the overheated child to shade and remove her or his clothing.

- Spray the child with cool water, and fan aggressively to increase evaporation. Cold packs may be applied to scalp, armpits, and the groin of very hot children.

- If the child is alert and not nauseated, give cool drinks to increase hydration.

Cold

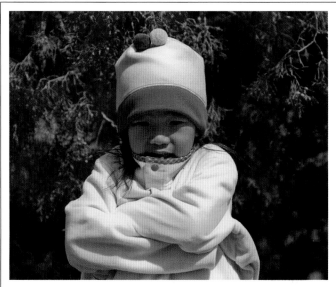

- Children who are too cold will shiver, move more slowly than usual, stumble, become uncoordinated, and slur their speech.

- Remove any damp clothing from the child and dress him or her in warm, dry clothing. Be sure the head and neck are covered. Hold the child close to you.

- For the very cold child, place heat packs on the chest, in the armpits, and on the neck.

- Give the alert child warm, sweet drinks.

not—"feel" cold as acutely as you. Insist on hats and mittens, and dress children in layers of clothing as you dress yourself (see "Preventing Hypothermia"). Children can overheat, just like you, on chilly days if dressed in too many layers. Layers can be taken off or put on.

Encourage your children to drink lots of water. And do not be surprised if they claim a lack of thirst. Children feel the need to drink less readily than adults. Thirst is often a sign that the body has already entered the early stages of dehydration. The old proverb advising "You can't drink too much water" is technically false but practically true. Water loss from your child can be significant during one hour of activity in a warm or cold climate. If you find it difficult to get kids to drink plain water, add enough powdered flavoring to make the water less boring but not enough to make it syrupy.

Hydration

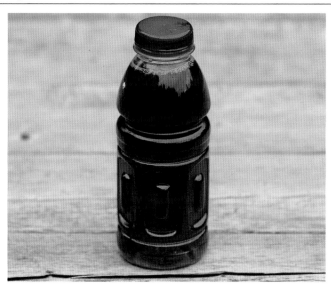

- Signs of dehydration in a child include thirst, dry lips, decreased and dark urine, and decreased tearing.

- Signs of severe dehydration include sunken eyes, loss of elasticity in the skin, and dry mouth and tongue (and a sunken fontanel in infants). Severe dehydration demands a physician as soon as possible.

- Treat dehydration by giving the child as much clear fluid as he or she will drink.

- Encourage hydration by supplying colorful clear fluids in colorful bottles.

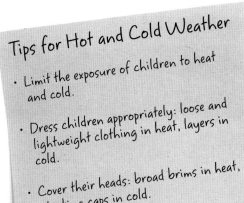

Tips for Hot and Cold Weather

- Limit the exposure of children to heat and cold.

- Dress children appropriately: loose and lightweight clothing in heat, layers in cold.

- Cover their heads: broad brims in heat, stocking caps in cold.

- Check in with children often.

INSECTS & CHILDREN
Bites and stings are generally a greater risk to kids than to adults

Children usually have more trouble than adults resisting the temptation to scratch itchy bites. Because children are also typically less hygienic than adults, scratches on children have a higher rate of infection. How you choose to prevent and treat bites is important.

Products that reduce the itching and, thus, the temptation to scratch are recommended. Use them as soon as possible after a bite. Hydrocortisone cream will reduce the itch of more established bites. To improvise an anti-itch medication, you may use a slurry of water and baking soda or meat tenderizer. Bites that are scratched open should be washed with soap and water and covered with an adhesive strip dressing.

For prevention, insect repellent should be used regularly. DEET, a common repelling ingredient, should not be used in a high concentration. For children, the lower the concentration, the better. Keep the repellent off children's hands, and

Repelling Insects

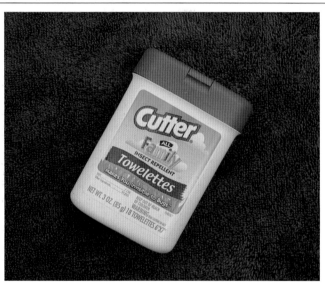

- Products that contain DEET repel mosquitoes best, and they also repel flies and ticks, but not quite as effectively.

- Some DEET is absorbed through skin, and a concentration of no more than 10 percent is recommended for children. You will have to reapply a 10 percent

concentration if exposure time is extended.

- DEET is poisonous if ingested and should always be stored out of reach of small children.

- Permethrin applied to clothing, but not skin, is a safe and effective repellent.

Applying Repellents

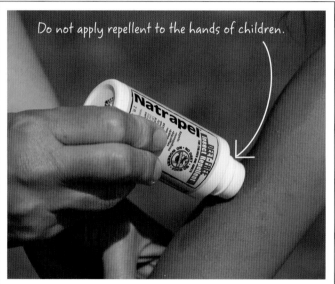

Do not apply repellent to the hands of children.

- Parents should apply repellents to small children instead of allowing children to apply it themselves. Keep it off their hands because they often rub it into their mouth and eyes.

- Apply repellents only to areas of exposed skin and

not to skin covered by clothing.

- Be sure to read the labels carefully on all products, and use such products only as directed.

- As soon as exposure has ended, wash repellents off.

you will reduce the chance that they will rub it into their eyes or, even worse, suck it off their fingers. You can avoid DEET by choosing products made with natural repellents, such as lemon eucalyptus oil (which has been proven as effective as approximately an 8 percent concentration of DEET). Other effective non-DEET repellents include those that use picaridin on skin and permethrin on clothing.

Fighting the Itch

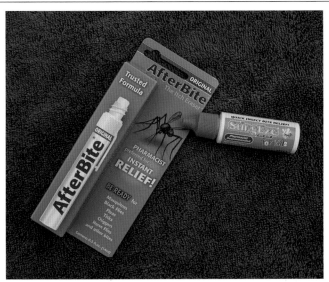

- Several commercial products effectively reduce the itch of insect bites and are safe to use on children.

- Itching can also be reduced by applying an ice cube or a cold, wet cloth.

- Sometimes a few moments of direct pressure on the bite with a clean fingernail or the cap of a pen will reduce the itching.

- For itching that resists these methods, a physician may recommend an oral antihistamine or a stronger anti-itch cream.

Serious Reactions

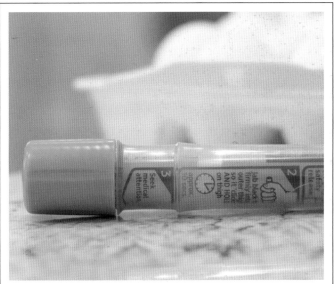

- More serious reactions to bites or stings often cause unusually large, firm swelling at the site and/or hives that typically appear on the trunk of the child (or adult).

- Abnormal reactions should be evaluated by a physician to determine if the child is severely allergic.

- The physician may prescribe an auto-injector of epinephrine in case of a life-threatening reaction.

- These auto-injectors are manufactured with a child-sized dose of the medication.

SUNLIGHT & CHILDREN
Direct ultraviolet light is more dangerous for kids than for adults

The sun is worse on kids than it is on adults, even though the damage may not show up for thirty years.

Children sunburn more easily than adults. Children should wear clothing woven tightly enough to protect their skin from ultraviolet light and hats with a brim to protect their faces.

Use sunscreen on unprotected skin. Ultraviolet A and B damage skin, and the sunscreen should protect against both.

Assume that the SPF (sun protection factor) is not as good as it claims, and use a higher number. Sunscreens should be applied in a uniform coat over all exposed areas. If children will be swimming, use a waterproof sunscreen, and reapply it often. A few inches of water will not protect your child's skin from sunburn. Once a pleasant suntan is established, the screen should still be used. Tans prevent burning but offer little protection from the harmful effects of the sun.

Sun Protection

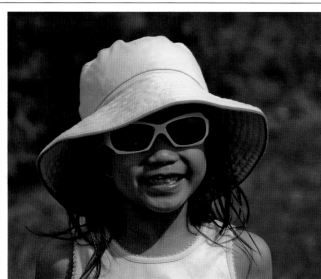

- Dress children in light-weight, light-colored clothing with a tight weave that covers as much of the skin as possible.

- Children should wear hats with a wide brim to protect their head, face, and neck. A floppy brim is more protective than a rigid brim.

- Children have the same need for sunglasses as adults. Wrap-around sunglasses provide better protection than flat sunglasses.

- A few manufacturers market children's clothing that is made to be especially protective.

Sunscreen

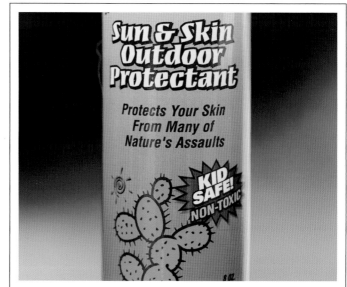

- Apply a sunscreen to areas of the child's skin that will be exposed to sunlight. But remember that sunscreen will burn if it gets into eyes.

- Use a product with an SPF of at least 15, and apply it thirty minutes prior to exposure to the sun.

- Be sure that the sunscreen protects against both ultraviolet A and ultraviolet B light.

- Reapply the sunscreen every three or four hours or right after swimming unless it is a waterproof product.

For young children, use a screen prepared as a milky lotion or cream, and avoid the upper and lower eyelids where the screen might be rubbed involuntarily into the eye. Never use baby oil in the sun.

Encourage children to wear sunglasses in order to reduce the chance of cataracts later in life and to protect their sensitive eyelids.

Cool compresses may reduce the pain and limit the depth of sunburn. Moisturizing lotions should be applied to skin. Acetaminophen may be given for pain. Drinking lots of water is important.

Limit Sun Exposure

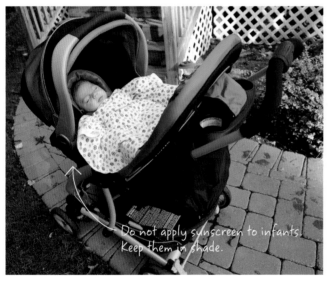

Do not apply sunscreen to infants. Keep them in shade.

- The damaging UV light of the sun reaches its peak between 10 A.M. and 3 P.M., hours when your child and you are most vulnerable. Limit your exposure during these hours.

- Ultraviolet light is reflected from sand, water, and snow.

- On an overcast day, approximately 70 percent of the sun's rays penetrate the clouds.

- Shade provided by a porch roof, a tree with dense foliage, and an umbrella is effective protection from the sun.

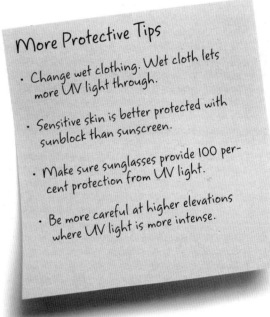

More Protective Tips

- Change wet clothing. Wet cloth lets more UV light through.

- Sensitive skin is better protected with sunblock than sunscreen.

- Make sure sunglasses provide 100 percent protection from UV light.

- Be more careful at higher elevations where UV light is more intense.

PEDIATRICS

ILLNESSES OF CHILDREN
Children get sick far more often than adults, but illness is usually not serious

As an average adult, you will have three or four illnesses per year, most of them minor. A child, on the other hand, will have six to eight, again, most of them minor. But you need to be able to recognize a more serious childhood illness.

Fevers are common in kids, and a fever is a strong indicator of the seriousness of an illness. To check for a fever in a child, leave the thermometer in an armpit for four minutes. An armpit temperature above 99°F is a fever. Leave a thermometer under the tongue for two or three minutes. An oral temperature greater than 100°F is a fever. Fevers greater than 102°F should send you to the doctor.

Monitor also the child's response to a fever. A child who

Colds

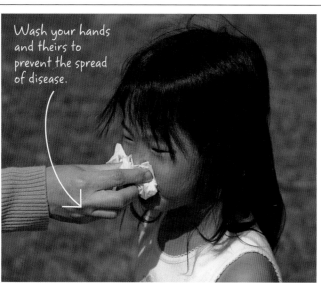

Wash your hands and theirs to prevent the spread of disease.

- During the first few days of a cold, children suffer runny noses, sore throats, and sometimes mild fevers, and they may say they feel "sick."

- After they feel better, you may notice an increase and thickening of nasal discharge.

- They often cough, especially at night.

- See a doctor if you think your child has a cold with an ear infection, an eye infection, a seriously sore throat, or a high fever.

Fever

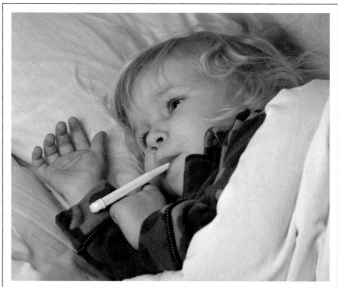

- The behavior of the child is more important than the degree of the fever.

- Find a doctor for children with a fever who also stare into space, refuse to smile, refuse to play, and are difficult to wake up.

- Find a doctor if the child complains of pain when touched, or if the child has labored breathing.

- Find a doctor if the child's temperature rises to 104°F or if a temperature of 102°F lasts for more than seventy-two hours.

behaves normally with a fever is less of a concern than a child who grows disinterested and lethargic.

Children with fevers need rest and plenty of fluids—but not aspirin. Acetaminophen may be given, preferably with a doctor's approval first.

Due to their shorter airways, children tend to have more difficulty breathing, and thus breathe more noisily, with illnesses of the upper respiratory system. If noisy breathing is persistent, and, of course, if it's severe, you should find a doctor.

Persistent diarrhea—several loose, watery stools per day—carries the risk of dehydration. Give plenty of clear fluids, and consider bland foods such as the BRAT diet: bananas, rice, applesauce, and toast. If the problem does not resolve within forty-eight hours, or if diarrhea is severe, consult a doctor.

Children vomit easily and fairly often, and it is seldom serious. With persistent vomiting, however, the child is at risk of dehydration and should be evaluated by a physician.

Treatment

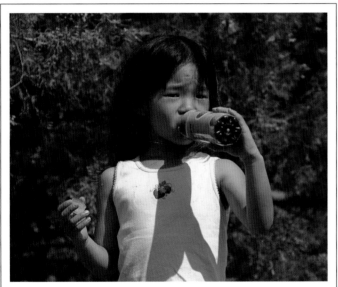

- Sick children need plenty of clear fluids—as much as you can get them to drink.

- Children mend best when they get plenty of rest as well.

- Children with a fever may be sponged lightly with lukewarm water if it makes them feel better.

- You may choose to give a medication for discomfort and fever, a child's dose of acetaminophen or ibuprofen, following the directions on the label and preferably after consulting your doctor.

More Warning Signs

- Breathing more than thirty times per minute

- Drooling or having the inability to swallow

- Having purple spots on the skin

- Having a stiff neck

- Having a bulging fontanel in infants

MEDICATIONS FOR CHILDREN

Kids sometimes cannot, and often should not, take the same medications as adults

Errors in giving medications to children are more likely to cause harm than errors in giving medications to adults. Children are less tolerant of many drugs and have adverse reactions to more drugs than do adults. In most cases, it is wisest to give no drugs to children without first consulting a physician.

Recommended doses of medications are based on the size of the body into which the medications are going. The medications for children you see over the counter are not just pretty colors and interesting flavors—the dose of the drug is based on the average size of the child. It is of the utmost importance to read and follow the directions on the labels.

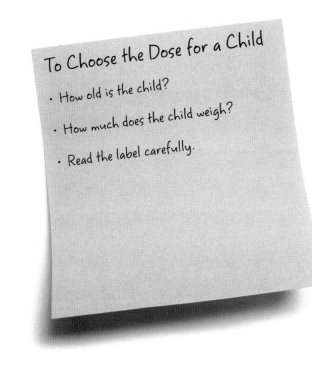

To Choose the Dose for a Child

- How old is the child?
- How much does the child weigh?
- Read the label carefully.

Medications

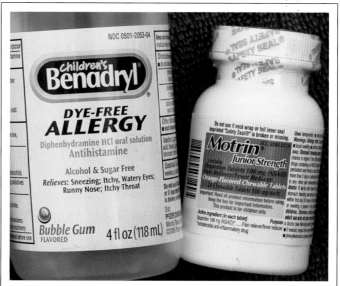

- Most children can handle chewable tablets after they get their first molars, at around fifteen months.

- Tablets can also be crushed between two spoons and added to food.

- Most medications for children are available in liquid form and/or in concentrated drops.

- In all cases, it is best to consult a physician prior to giving any medication to a child the first time. Consider the consultation prior to needing to give the medication.

Children aged five and under usually cannot swallow pills. Use chewable tablets. For children too little to chew, the tablets can be crushed and added to food. Or choose medications in liquid form.

In emergency situations where a physician is not readily available, it is usually safe to give child-strength acetaminophen and/or ibuprofen for pain and/or fever. Child-strength antihistamines are usually safe as well. In all cases, it is best to consult your family doctor before an emergency arises.

Aspirin

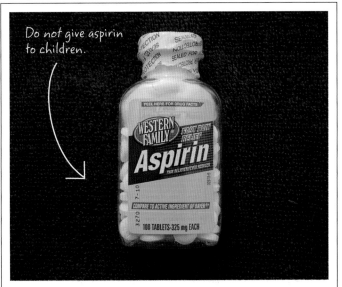

Do not give aspirin to children.

- Children sixteen years of age and younger should *not* be given aspirin for any reason.

- Aspirin may precipitate a potentially fatal illness called "Reye's syndrome" that causes the brain to swell.

- The syndrome is indicated by heavy vomiting, lethargy, and confusion, followed by stupor and hyperventilation and then coma.

- A child suspected of having Reye's syndrome must be transported to a hospital with the greatest possible speed.

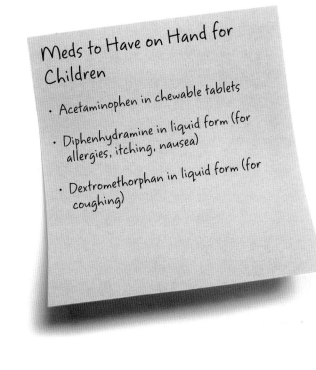

Meds to Have on Hand for Children

- Acetaminophen in chewable tablets

- Diphenhydramine in liquid form (for allergies, itching, nausea)

- Dextromethorphan in liquid form (for coughing)

PEDIATRICS

GRIEF, ANXIETY, & PANIC
Emotional responses to loss, apprehension, and fear can trigger different responses in different people

Grief is the emotional response to loss, and even something as simple as permanently losing your favorite book can generate a small degree of grief. Sorrow and regret can be sharp and painful in times of major loss. It is not unusual for someone to cry easily or express apparently unexplained sadness when that person is in mourning. Identifying the cause of the grieving

behavior might well be a relief for everyone concerned.

If a person must be told that someone close has just died, be prepared for any behavior. Some people lash out, and others draw within, just as in any other personal crisis. It is best to hear the news from someone whom that person knows well.

Stages of the Grieving Process

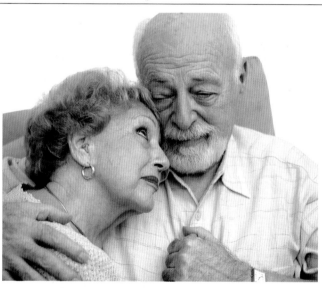

- A "grief spike" that lasts from five to fifteen minutes

- A period of denial

- A period of anger and guilty feelings

- A period of depression

- Acceptance

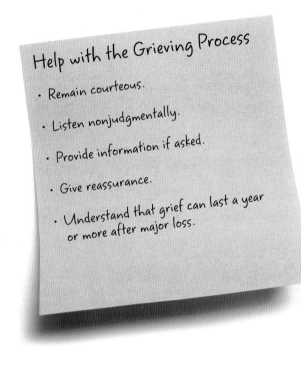

Help with the Grieving Process

- Remain courteous.

- Listen nonjudgmentally.

- Provide information if asked.

- Give reassurance.

- Understand that grief can last a year or more after major loss.

Acute anxiety or panic attacks are characterized by a discrete but predictable onset of symptoms, often without an apparent cause. Physical signs and symptoms may include rapid heartbeat or palpitations, light-headedness and/or dizziness, sweating, trembling, and shaking, perhaps associated with hot flashes or cold chills and tingling in the fingers or toes. There are often overwhelming feelings of terror or apprehension and fear of dying, losing control, or "going crazy." Your intervention can be extremely beneficial. People with recurring or persistent anxiety or panic require the intervention of a professional.

Recognizing a Panic Attack

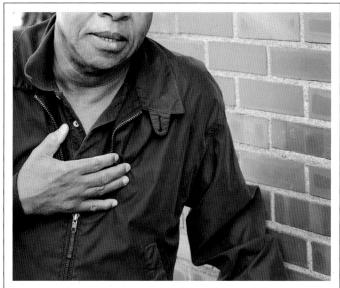

- Rapid heartbeat

- Light-headedness or dizziness

- Sweating, shaking, sometimes fainting

- Feelings of terror and/or apprehension

- Feelings of loss of control

- Inexplicable fear of dying

YELLOW LIGHT

If someone with the described symptoms has not lost touch with reality, the cause is likely to be a panic disorder. For those who have lost touch with reality, there may be an affective disorder or organic cause. Other conditions associated with anxiety and panic include phobias, hyperventilation syndrome, and generalized anxiety disorder (characterized by persistent anxiety of at least a month-long duration).

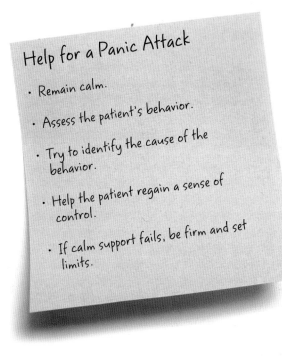

Help for a Panic Attack

- Remain calm.

- Assess the patient's behavior.

- Try to identify the cause of the behavior.

- Help the patient regain a sense of control.

- If calm support fails, be firm and set limits.

PSYCHOLOGICAL, BEHAVIORAL

DEPRESSION & SUICIDAL BEHAVIOR

Clinical depression is enduring and can lead to thoughts of suicide

Feeling depressed, to some degree and in varying lengths of time, is common to almost everyone. This is normal, and the feelings pass. Clinical depression is different because it is enduring. Depression is known as an "affective disorder." This means it is outwardly manifested by mood, feelings, or tone, in this case characterized by lowered or diminished actions and feelings.

Anyone who speaks of suicide or makes suicidal gestures should be taken seriously. It may seem difficult to broach the subject, but if suicidal thoughts are suspected, inquire directly. If a person who was previously considering suicide seems suddenly better emotionally and behaviorally, the "miraculous" recovery may instead mean a decision has been made to go through with it. The patient may feel that the conflict has been taken out of the situation.

Recognizing Depression

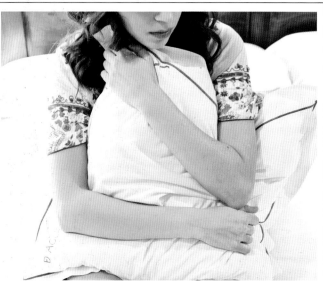

- Enduring irritability, sadness, or hopelessness

- Too much or too little sleep

- Eating disorders with weight loss or gain

- Loss of interest or pleasure

- Loss of energy and unusual fatigue

- Poor self-care

Help for the Depressed Person

- Talk about the problem with the person.

- Be honest and direct.

- Listen nonjudgmentally.

- Encourage adequate rest and nutrition.

- Seek professional assistance.

Two criteria are needed for identification of clinical depression: (1) a mood characterized by feeling blue, irritable, hopeless, depressed, or sad and (2) at least four of the following symptoms present almost continuously for at least two weeks:
1. Sleep disturbance (too much or too little)
2. Eating disorder with significant weight loss or gain
3. Psychomotor agitation or retardation
4. Loss of interest or pleasure in usual activities
5. Fatigue and loss of energy
6. Feelings of worthlessness and guilt
7. Difficulty concentrating or paying attention
8. Preoccupying thoughts of death or suicidal feelings

Symptoms of Suicidal Behavior

- Showing signs and symptoms of depression

- Feeling loss of interest in usual activities

- Speaking of suicide

- Making suicidal gestures

Dealing with a Suicidal Person

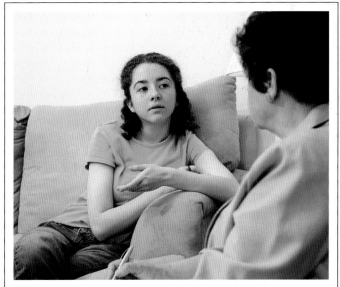

- Treat the patient normally.

- Let the patient talk.

- Use questions that require thoughtful answers.

- Avoid judgmental or opinionated replies.

- Seek professional help.

PSYCHOLOGICAL, BEHAVIORAL

MANIA & ASSAULTIVE BEHAVIOR

Hyperactive and aggressive individuals can be extremely difficult to be around

Mania is a mood disorder characterized by excessive elation, agitation and irritability, accelerated speaking, hyperactivity, and sometimes unusual thought patterns. Ideas may flood out so fast that none seems connected with the next, a phenomenon known as a "flight of ideas." The patient often displays poor judgment and provocative or intrusive behavior.

Mania may induce a decreased need for sleep and exaggerated feelings of power or capability. A manic person can be extremely difficult to be around, especially if you do not understand the nature of the disorder.

Mania ranges from mild to full-blown with hallucinations and delusions. Sometimes mania and depression combine in a

Symptoms of Mania

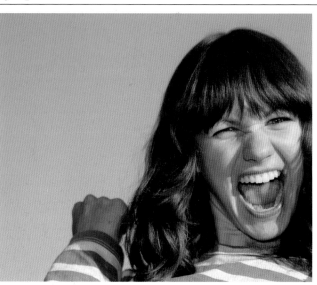

- Excessive elation and agitation
- Accelerated speaking
- Hyperactivity
- Displays of poor judgment
- Decreased need for sleep
- Mania can be caused by drug abuse and brain tumors. In all cases, persons with severe manic disorder require the intervention of a professional.

Dealing with a Manic Person

- Stay calm.
- Talk about what you observe.
- Avoid confrontation.
- Do not attempt to manhandle the person.
- Seek professional assistance.

cyclical pattern known as "bipolar disease." A person with such a disease experiences extreme and uncontrollable mood swings from the depressed end of the spectrum to the manic.

For many reasons, people sometimes become menacing or assaultive. In a time of crisis, people typically rely on old behavioral patterns for survival. Those who become aggressive may act on those feelings and become physically dangerous to others.

Resolving such a situation requires good rapport and tact. The goal is to calm the individual, not to trigger worse behavior. In some cases, it may be best not to intervene until later. At other times, someone who is out of control may need physical restraint. Evidence of homicidal intentions, for example, should be treated seriously and immediately. When enough people are available, use all the resources available, and coordinate the effort through good communication. One person per extremity is best—hold the elbows and knees, not the feet and hands. Let restraint accomplish its intended purposes without seeming punitive or brutal.

Symptoms of Assaultive Behavior

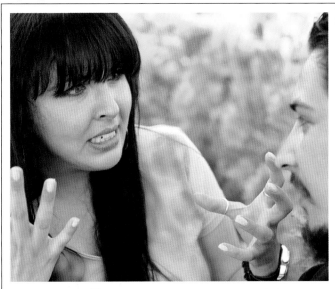

- Expressions of frustration and/or hostility

- Socially unacceptable activity

- Expressions of turbulent thoughts and/or feelings

- Destructive activity

- Excessively assaultive behavior and anyone who requires restraint should be evaluated by a professional

Resolving an Assaultive Situation

- If possible, wait until the crisis passes before confronting the patient.

- Use tact, establish good rapport.

- Calm the individual.

- Avoid triggering worse behavior.

- Use restraint only to prevent harm to yourself or others.

FIRST-AID KITS
Choose and maintain your kit

Generally speaking, better tools make better carpenters, and, likewise, better first-aid kits make better first-aid providers. That said, here are a few things to think about when you choose and maintain a first-aid kit:

1. Unfortunately, there is no perfect first-aid kit. No matter how much you plan and prepare, someday you will want something that is not there and/or discover you've had an item in your kit for years and never used it. When considering the contents of a kit, take into account (a) the number of people who might use your kit; (b) your distance from definitive medical care; (c) the availability of rescue, such as an ambulance; (d) your medical expertise; and (e) existing medical conditions in you and your family.

2. Evaluate and repack your kit regularly. Add the things you wish you had had last time. Renew medications that have reached expiration dates. Replace items that have been damaged by heat, cold, or moisture. Replace items you used.

3. Do not fill your kit with items you do not know how to use. Maintain a high level of familiarity with the proper uses of all the items in your kit.

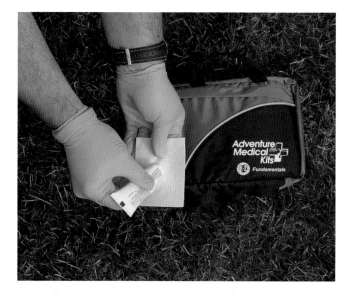

4. Know where your kit is at all times.

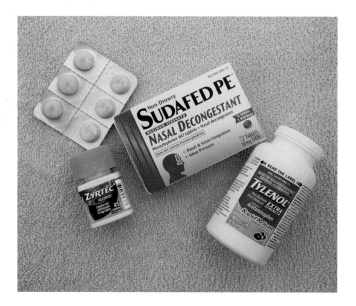

Specific considerations for your kit

Specific considerations for what to include in your kit can be divided into four categories: injury management supplies, tools, miscellaneous supplies, and medications. Keep in mind that these are suggestions and not requirements.

Injury Management Supplies to Consider

- ❑ Adhesive strip bandages
- ❑ Sterile gauze pads and/or sterile gauze rolls
- ❑ Athletic tape, 1 inch by 10 yards, and/or duct tape
- ❑ Tincture of benzoin compound
- ❑ Wound closure strips
- ❑ Microthin film dressings
- ❑ Large trauma dressings
- ❑ Moleskin and/or molefoam
- ❑ Gel wound/burn coverings
- ❑ Antimicrobial towelettes and/or alcohol wipes
- ❑ Lightweight splint
- ❑ Elastic wraps
- ❑ Protective medical gloves

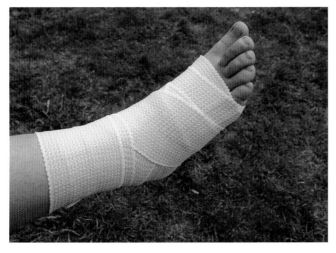

Tools to Consider

- ❑ Trauma shears
- ❑ Forceps (tweezers)
- ❑ Irrigation syringe
- ❑ Disposable scalpels
- ❑ Safety pins

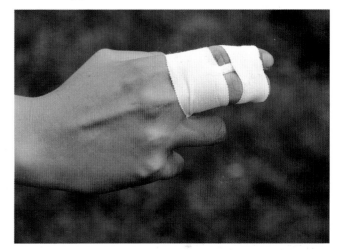

Miscellaneous Supplies to Consider

- ❑ Pad and pencil
- ❑ Pocket rescue mask
- ❑ Thermometer

Medications to Consider

- ❑ Nonsteroidal anti-inflammatory drugs
- ❑ Antacids
- ❑ Decongestants
- ❑ Antihistamines

Note: Consult your physician concerning drugs that should be kept on hand at all times.

FIRST-AID MATERIALS

Sources of Training

American Heart Association National Center, 7272 Greenville Avenue, Dallas, TX 75231. (800) 242-8721. www.americanheart.org.

American Red Cross National Headquarters, 2025 E Street NW, Washington, DC 20006. (202) 303-5000. www.redcross.org.

National Safety Council, 1121 Spring Lake Drive, Itasca, IL 60143. (800) 621-7615. www.nsc.org.

Sources of Information

American Academy of Orthopaedic Surgeons, 6300 North River Road, Rosemont, IL 60018. (847) 823-7186. www.aaos.org.

American Academy of Pediatrics, 141 Northwest Point Boulevard, Elk Grove Village, IL 60007. (847) 434-4000. www.aap.org.

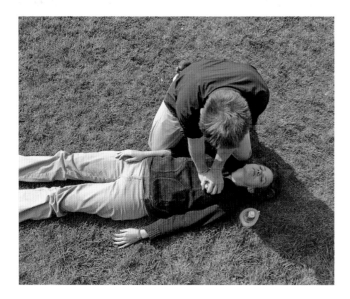

American Association of Poison Control Centers. (800) 222-1222. www.aapcc.org.

American Diabetes Association, 1701 North Beauregard Street, Alexandria, VA 22311. (800) 342-2383. www.diabetes.org.

American Heart Association National Center, 7272 Greenville Avenue, Dallas, TX 75231. (800) 242-8721. www.americanheart.org.

American Lung Association National Headquarters, 1301 Pennsylvania Avenue NW, Suite 800, Washington, DC 20004. (212) 315-8700. www.lungusa.org.

American Red Cross National Headquarters, 2025 E Street NW, Washington, DC 20006. (202) 303-5000. www.redcross.org.

American Stroke Association National Center, 7272 Greenville Avenue, Dallas, TX 75231. (888) 478-7653. www.strokeassociation.org.

Asthma and Allergy Foundation of America, 1233 20th Street NW, Suite 402, Washington, DC 20036. (800) 727-8462. www.aafa.org.

Centers for Disease Control and Prevention, 1600 Clifton Road, Atlanta, GA 30333. (800) 232-4636. www.cdc.gov.

Institute for Altitude Medicine, 500 West Pacific Avenue, Telluride, CO 81435. (970) 728-6767. http://altitudemedicine.org.

National Safety Council, 1121 Spring Lake Drive, Itasca, IL 60143. (800) 621-7615. www.nsc.org.

United States Army Research Institute of Environmental Medicine, Public Affairs Office, Kansas Street, Building 42, Natick, MA 01760. www.usariem.army.mil.

Books

AMA. *American Medical Association Handbook of First Aid and Emergency Care*. New York: Random House, 2000.

DK Publishing. *American College of Emergency Physicians First Aid Manual*. New York: Dorling Kindersley Limited, 2002.

Forgey, William. *Basic Essentials Hypothermia*. Guilford, CT: The Globe Pequot Press, 1999.

Handal, Kathleen A. *The American Red Cross First Aid and Safety Handbook*. Washington, DC: American Red Cross, 1992.

Kavanagh, James. *Emergency First Aid*. Guilford, CT: Waterford Press, 2001.

Tilton, Buck. *Backcountry First Aid & Extended Care, Fifth Edition*. Guilford, CT: The Globe Pequot Press, 2007.

Tilton, Buck. *Wilderness First Responder, Third Edition*. Guilford, CT: The Globe Pequot Press, 2010.

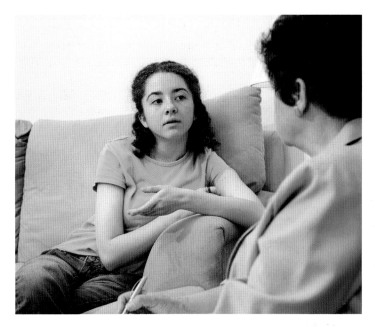

GLOSSARY

A

Abduction: Movement away from the midline of the body.

Abrasion: Wound in which one or more layers of skin are scraped away.

Acclimatization: Process of physiologically adjusting to a new environment, e.g., altitude.

Acute: An immediate problem with a short duration; not chronic.

Acute Mountain Sickness (AMS): Non-specific problems caused by a failure to acclimatize to higher altitudes; the first stage in a progression that can lead to H.A.C.E.

Adduction: Movement toward the midline of the body

Allergen: Allergy-causing substance.

Alveoli: Microscopic sacs of the lungs where gas exchange takes place.

Ambulatory: Able to walk.

Amenorrhea: Absence of a menstrual cycle.

Amnesia: Loss of memory.

Amniotic Sac: Thin membrane covering the fetus and placenta and containing amniotic fluid.

Amputation: A separation of a body part from the rest of the body.

Analgesic: Pain reliever.

Anaphylaxis: Severe allergic reaction to a foreign protein characterized by bronchoconstriction and vasodilation.

Anesthetic: Agent that produces a partial or complete loss of sensation.

Angina Pectoris: Pain in the chest caused by the heart demanding more blood than is available via the coronary circulation.

Anorexia: Loss of appetite.

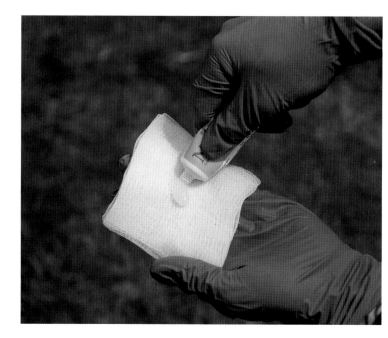

Anovulatory Cycle: No ovulation.

Anterior: Front surface.

Antibiotic: Substance that inhibits growth of or destroys microorganisms.

Antiemetic: Substance used to prevent or treat vomiting.

Antihistamine: Drug that counteracts the effects of histamines.

Anti-inflammatory: Substance used to counteract inflammation.

Antipyretic: Agent that reduces or relieves fever.

Antivenin: Serum containing antitoxin for a venom.

Aorta: Main artery that leaves the heart and travels to the body.

Apnea: Absence of breathing.

Appendicitis: Inflammation of the appendix.

Arteriole: Small artery.

Arteriosclerosis: Thickening, hardening, and loss of elasticity of the arteries.

Artery: Vessel carrying blood from the heart.

Asphyxia: Condition of insufficient intake of oxygen.

Aspirate: To draw in or out by suction; to inhale particulate matter.

Asthma: Condition resulting in shortness of breath and wheezing due to swelling of bronchi and swelling of their mucous membranes.

Asystole: Absence of all activity in the heart.

Ataxia: Loss of muscle coordination leading to difficulty in maintaining balance.

Atherosclerosis: Clogging of the arteries from fatty deposits and other debris.

Auscultate: Listen.

Avulsion: Forcible tearing away of a part or structure; a piece of skin left hanging as a flap.

Axial: The imaginary line through the middle of the body, or through the middle of a part of the body.

B

Bacteria: Single-cell microorganisms.

Basal Metabolic Rate (BMR): The constant rate at which a human body consumes energy to drive chemical reactions and produce heat to maintain an adequate core temperature at rest.

Battle's Sign: Bruising behind and below the ears indicating a fracture to the base of the skull.

Bipolar Disease: Cyclical pattern of depression and mania.

Bleb: Fluid-filled blister.

Brachial: Arm from the shoulder to the elbow.

Bradycardia: Slow heart rate.

Breech Presentation: Baby presents feet or buttocks first during birth.

Bronchiole: Small airway of the lung.

Bronchitis: Inflammation of the mucous membranes of the bronchi.

Bronchospasm: Spasms in the muscles of the bronchi.

Bronchus: One of the two large airways branching off from the trachea.

Bursae: Fluid-filled sac or cavity commonly found in joints.

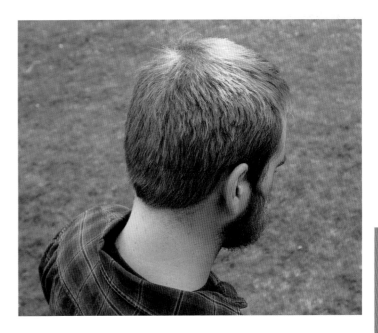

C

Calcaneous: Heel bone.

Capillary: Minute blood vessel where gas exchange occurs between the bloodstream and the tissues.

Cardiac Arrest: The cessation of useful heart muscle activity.

Cardiogenic: Originating in the heart.

Cardiovascular System: Relating to the heart, the blood vessels, and the blood.

Carotid Artery: Primary blood vessel supplying the head and neck of which there are two.

Carpopedal Spasms: Muscular spasms in the hands and feet.

Cartilage: Tough elastic tissue forming protective pads where bone meets bone.

Cerebellum: Part of the brain that helps control movement and balance.

Cerebral: Relating to the cerebrum.

Cerebrovascular Accident (CVA): Interruption of normal blood flow to a part of the brain; stroke.

Cerebrum: Largest part of the brain, it consists of two hemispheres.

Cervical Vertebrae: First seven bones of the spinal column; the neck bones.

Cervix: Narrow opening at the low end of the uterus.

Chronic: Slow progression or of long duration; not acute.

Chronic Obstructive Pulmonary Disease (COPD): A collection of diseases sharing the common symptoms of airway obstruction in the small to medium airways, excessive secretions, and/or constriction of the bronchial tubes.

Clavicle: Collarbone.

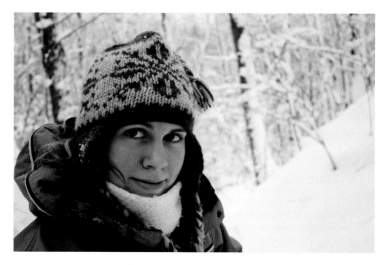

Closed Pneumothorax: Tear in the lining of the lung resulting in air accumulating in the pleural space with no open wounds.

Coma: An unconsciousness level from which the patient cannot be aroused.

Comminuted Fracture: Fracture in which the bone is splintered or crushed.

Conduction: Heat lost from a warmer object when it comes in contact with a colder object.

Congestive Heart Failure (CHF): Condition in which blood and tissue fluids congest due to the heart's inadequacy.

Conjunctiva: Membrane lining the eyes.

Constipation: Infrequent or difficult bowel movements.

Contusion: Bruise.

Convection: Heat lost directly into air or water by movement.

Coronary Artery: Vessel that supplies the heart muscle with blood.

Cranium: Skull.

Crepitus: Sound or feel of broken bone ends grating against each other.

Cyanosis: Blue hue to the skin indicating a lack of oxygen in the blood.

D

Defibrillation: Stopping fibrillation of the heart using electricity or drugs.

Depression: Altered mood characterized by lack of interest in pleasurable things.

Dermatitis: Inflammation of the skin.

Dermis: True skin.

Diabetes Mellitus: Disease in which the pancreas secretes an insufficient or ineffective amount of insulin.

Diaphoresis: Profuse sweating.

Diaphragm: Large muscle separating the abdominal and thoracic cavities; the primary muscle used in breathing.

Dislocation: The complete or partial disruption of the normal relationship of a joint.

Distal: Away from the center.

Diuretic: Drug that causes increased urination.

Dysentery: Bacterially caused diarrhea that may produce blood and mucus in the stool.

Dysmenorrhea: Pain associated with menstruation.

Dyspnea: Difficulty breathing.

E

Ecchymosis: Bruising.

Ectopic Pregnancy: Pregnancy that implants outside of the uterus, commonly in a fallopian tube.

Edema: Swelling from too much fluid.

Efface: Thin, as in the cervix during labor.

Embolism: Obstruction of a blood vessel by a clot of blood or a foreign substance.

Emesis: Vomit.

Emetics: Vomit inducers.

Emphysema: Chronic pulmonary disease characterized by destruction of the alveoli.

Endometrium: Lining of the uterus.

Envenomation: Introduction of poison into the body by a bite or sting.

Epidermis: Thin outer layer of the skin.

Epididymis: Organ lying behind the testicle that stores sperm.

Epididymitis: Inflammation of the epididymis.

Epigastric: Upper abdomen.

Epiglottis: Structure overlying the larynx that prevents food or liquid from entering the airway during swallowing.

Epistaxis: Nosebleed.

Eschar: Scab.

Esophagus: Tube carrying food and liquid from the mouth to the stomach.

Eustachian Tube: Tube extending from the middle ear to the back of the throat.

Evaporation: The process in which a liquid changes into vapor.

Eversion: Turning outward.

Evisceration: Abdominal contents exposed and protruding from an open wound.

Exhalation: Breathing out.

F

Fallopian Tube: Tube extending from the ovary to the uterus.

Fascia: Membrane that covers muscle.

Febrile: Feverish.

Fecal Impaction: Hardened feces forming a blockage in the descending colon preventing passage of fecal material.

Femoral: Relating to the femur.

Femur: Thigh bone.

Fibrin: Protein that forms a matrix for clotting and scabbing.

Fibula: Small lower leg bone.

Flail Chest: Two or more ribs fractured in two or more places creating a floating section of rib.

Fracture: A break in the normal continuity of a bone.

Frostbite: Localized tissue damage caused by freezing.

Frostnip: Superficial frostbite.

Fungus: Primitive life form that feeds on living plants, decaying organic matter, and animal tissue.

G

Gallstone: Concretion formed in the gallbladder or bile duct.

Gastric Distention: Air overinflating the stomach.

Gastritis: Inflammation of the stomach.

Gastrocolic: Relating to the stomach and colon.

Gastroenteritis: Inflammation of the gastrointestinal tract.

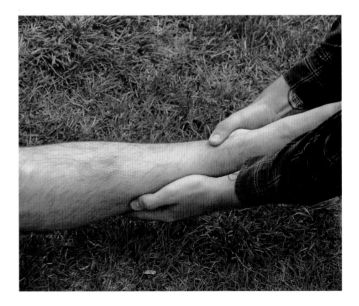

Germ: Microscopic organism that might infect a human and cause disease.

Glottis: The vocal cords and space between them at the opening of the trachea.

Glucagon: Hormone that increases the concentration of glucose in the blood.

Gluteals: Muscles of the buttocks.

Greenstick Fracture: Fracture that does not extend all the way through the bone.

Grief: Emotional response to loss.

Gross Negligence: Extreme deviation from the accepted standard of care.

Guarding: Protecting an area of injury through muscle tension and/or physical positioning.

H

Hamstrings: Muscles in the back of the upper leg.

Heat Cramps: Painful spasm of major muscles being exercised, caused by dehydration in association with electrolyte depletion.

Heat Exhaustion: Weakness produced by fluid loss from excessive sweating in a hot environment that causes compensatory shock.

Heat Stroke: Life-threatening condition produced by exposure to hot environments and/or excessive heat production described by an elevated core temperature that causes the brain to "cook."

Hematemesis: Blood in the vomit.

Hematoma: Pooling of blood in the form of a tumor.

Hematuria: Blood in the urine.

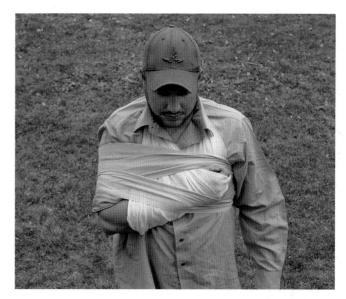

Hemiparesis: Weakness affecting one side of the body.

Hemiplegia: Paralysis affecting one side of the body.

Hemoptysis: Coughing up blood.

Hemorrhage: Bleeding.

Hemostasis: Control of bleeding.

Hemothorax: Blood in the pleural space.

High Altitude Cerebral Edema (H.A.C.E.): Fluid collecting in the patient's brain as a result of extremes of elevation gain.

High Altitude Pulmonary Edema (H.A.P.E.): Fluid shifting from the pulmonary capillaries and filling the alveolar spaces as a result of extremes of elevation gain.

Histamine: Natural substance in the body released by the immune system in response to an injury or foreign protein.

Humerus: Upper arm bone.

Hymenoptera: Bees, wasps, and fire ants.

Hyperglycemia: High blood sugar.

Hypertension: High blood pressure.

Hyperventilation: Breathing unusually fast and/or deep.

Hyperventilation Syndrome: Breathing fast and deep without another cause.

Hypoglycemia: Low blood sugar.

Hypostome: Feeding apparatus of a tick.

Hypotension: Lowered blood pressure.

Hypothalamus: A structure in the brain responsible for controlling certain metabolic activities including temperature regulation.

Hypothermia: Lowered core temperature.

Hypovolemic: Low blood volume.

Hypoxia: Low oxygen level.

I

Immersion Foot: A nonfreezing cold injury from prolonged contact with cold and, typically, moisture that causes inadequate circulation and tissue damage.

Impacted Fracture: Fracture in which broken bone ends are wedged together.

Implied Consent: Legal assumption that an unconscious and/or unreliable patient would desire treatment if they were conscious or reliable enough to make a decision. Also applies to minors when a parent or guardian is unavailable to offer consent.

Incision: Smooth-edged cut through the skin made by a sharp edge.

Incontinence: Loss of bowel and/or bladder control.

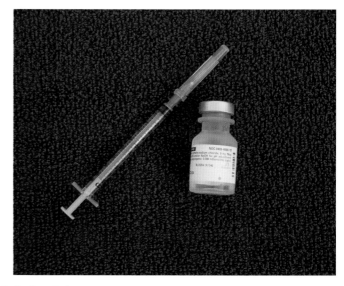

Inferior: Below.

Inflammation: Successive changes in tissue in response to injury.

Informed Consent: Consent to treat obtained from a patient who has been informed of the potential risks and benefits of a proposed treatment.

Inguinal Hernia: A hernia in the region of the groin.

Inhalation: Breathing in.

Insomnia: Inability to sleep.

Insulin: Hormone required to move glucose out of the bloodstream and through cell walls that is manufactured in the pancreas.

Integumentary System: Skin.

Intercostal Muscles: Muscles between the ribs.

Inversion: Turning inward.

Ischemia: Lack of blood supply.

K

Keratin: Hard protein in skin, nails, and hair.

Kidney Stone: Concretion formed in the kidney and excreted through the urinary tract.

L

Laceration: An irregular cut or tear through the skin.

Lacrimal: Relating to tears.

Laryngospasm: A constrictive spasm of the muscles of the upper airway.

Larynx: Structure of cartilage that holds open the upper end of the trachea; the "voice box."

Lassitude: Weariness, exhaustion.

Lateral: Away from the midline of the body; the outer aspect.

Lesion: An area of pathologically altered tissue; a wound or injury.

Ligament: Connective tissue holding bone to bone.

Lumbar Vertebrae: Five bones of the lower spine found between the thoracic vertebrae and the sacrum.

Lymphadentitis: Inflammation of the lymph nodes.

Lymphangitis: Inflammation of the lymph channels or vessels.

M

Malaise: General feeling of discomfort or indisposition.

Malleolus: Rounded distal end of the tibia or fibula; the "ankle bones."

Mania: Mood disorder characterized by excessive elation, agitation, accelerated speaking, and hyperactivity.

Medial: Near the midline; the inner aspect.

Medulla: Lower portion of the brain stem.

Menarche: Initial menstrual period.

Meninges: Three membranes surrounding the brain and spinal cord—the dura mater, the arachnoid, and the pia mater.

Meniscus: Crescent-shaped fibrocartilage in the knee joint.

Miscarriage: Spontaneous abortion.

Mittelschmerz: Pain associated with ovulation.

Mucus: Viscous fluid secreted by the mucous membranes.

Mucous Membranes: Membranes that line passages and cavities communicating with the air.

Myocardial Infarction: Death of a portion of the heart muscle resulting from a blockage in the coronary circulation; a heart attack.

Myocardium: Heart muscle.

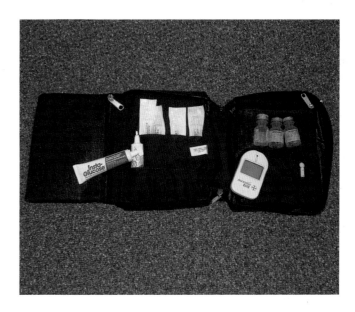

N

Nasopharynx: Posterior part of the nose; the part of the pharynx above the soft palate.

Necrosis: Tissue death.

Negligence: The careless, unintentional act that harms another person to whom you owe a duty of care.

Neurogenic: Originating in the nervous tissue.

O

Open Fracture: Any fracture over which the skin is broken.

Open Pneumothorax: Open wound causing a tear in the lining of the lung resulting in air accumulating in the pleural space.

Ophthalmic: Relating to the eye.

Oropharynx: Posterior part of the mouth; the part of the pharynx between the soft palate and the epiglottis.

Ovary: Gland that produces eggs in the female reproductive system.

Ovulation: Release of an egg from an ovary.

Ovum: Egg.

P

Palliate: To reduce pain or make feel better.

Palpate: To feel by touching.

Paradoxical Respirations: Asymmetrical chest wall movement associated with a flail chest.

Paraparesis: Partial paralysis of the lower portion of the body.

Paraplegia: Paralysis of the lower portion of the body.

Parasite: Organism that lives on or within another organism.

Paresthesia: Loss of or unusual sensations; "pins and needles."

Patella: Kneecap.

Patent: Clear and open, as in an airway.

Pathogen: Microorganism capable of producing disease.

Pathological: Concerning disease.

Pedal: Relating to the foot.

Perfusion: Fluid, typically well-oxygenated blood, passing through an organ or tissue.

Pericardial Sac: Sac surrounding the heart.

Perineal: Region of the vagina and anus.

Peripheral: Away from the center; near the edge.

Peritonitis: Inflammation of the abdominal lining (peritoneum).

Permethrin: Insect repellent spray applied to clothing; an insecticide.

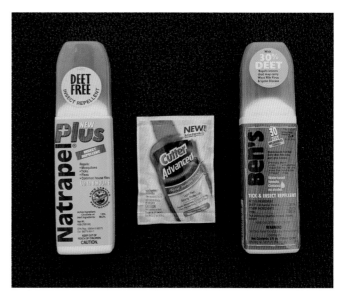

Placenta: Organ that provides nourishment to the fetus.

Placenta Previa: A placenta that implants over the cervix.

Placental Abruption: Separation of the placenta from the uterine wall.

Pleura: Membrane that surrounds both lungs and extends to line the chest cavity.

Pneumonia: Infection or inflammation in the lungs.

Pneumonic: Concerning the lungs.

Pneumothorax: Tear in the lining of the lung resulting in air accumulating in the pleural space.

Polyuria: Increased volume of urine output.

Posterior: Back surface.

Postictal: Period of recovery following a seizure.

Premenstrual Syndrome (PMS): Cluster of symptoms that occur prior to menstruation.

Prolapsed Cord: A presentation of the umbilical cord in the vaginal canal prior to the baby.

Prone: Face down.

Proximal: Nearest the midline of the body; nearest the center.

Psychogenic: Originating in the mind.

Pulmonary Edema: Fluid in the lungs.

Pulmonary Embolism: Blockage in a pulmonary artery or arteriole.

Puncture: Wound made by a pointed object such as knife, bullet, or ice axe.

Q

Quadriceps: Thigh muscles.

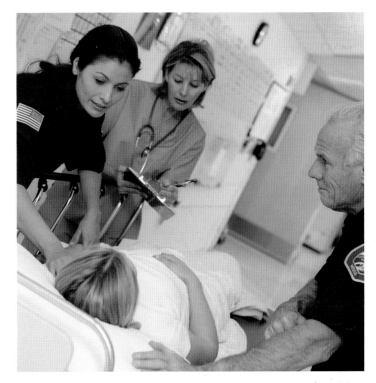

Quadriplegia: Paralysis of all four extremities.

R

Raccoon Eyes: Bruising around the eyes, indicative of a skull fracture.

Radial: Pertaining to the radius.

Radiation: Heat given off by a warm object.

Radius: Shorter lower arm bone.

Reduction: A return to normal anatomical relationship.

Respiratory Arrest: Cessation of breathing.

S

Sacrum: Five fused bones of vertebrae between the lumbar spine and the coccyx; one of three bones of the pelvic ring.

Scapula: Shoulder blade.

Scrotum: Sac containing the testicles and some other parts of the reproductive system in males.

Seizure: A sudden, abnormal electrical discharge in the brain.

Separation: Enlargement of the spaces between bones.

Sepsis: Illness resulting from a buildup of microorganisms or their toxins in the blood.

Septicemia: "Blood poisoning" from buildup of bacteria or their toxins in the blood.

Serum: The watery portion of blood.

Shin: Front of the lower leg.

Spontaneous Pneumothorax: Tear in the lining of the lung resulting in air accumulating in the pleural space that occurs without trauma.

Sprain: Stretching or tearing of ligaments.

Sputum: Substance coughed up from the airway.

Sternum: Breastbone.

Strain: Stretching or tearing of muscle fibers or tendons.

Stridor: High-pitched sound created by constrictions in the airway.

Subcutaneous: Under the skin.

Sucking Chest Wound: Open pneumothorax.

Superior: Above.

Supine: Face up.

Syncope: Fainting.

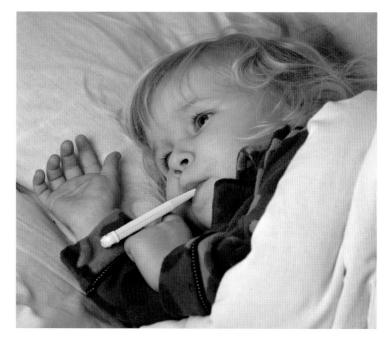

T

Tachycardia: Rapid heart rate.

Talus: The true ankle bone.

Tendinitis: Inflammation of a tendon, also spelled tendonitis.

Tendon: Connective tissue holding muscle to bone.

Tension Pneumothorax: Buildup of air in the pleural space that collapses the injured lung and begins to exert pressure on the uninjured lung and the heart.

Testis: Gland that produces sperm; testicle, gonad.

Tetanic Contraction: Continuous uterine contraction.

Thermoregulation: Body core temperature regulation.

Thoracic Vertebrae: The twelve vertebrae between the cervical vertebrae and the lumbar vertebrae with ribs attached on both sides.

Thorax: Chest cavity.

Tibia: Large lower leg bone.

Torsion of the Testis: Twisting of the testis on the spermatic cord.

Trachea: Windpipe.

Transient Ischemic Attack (TIA): Temporary stroke with signs and symptoms lasting less than twenty-four hours.

Transverse Fracture: Horizontal break in a bone.

Tumor: A swelling or enlargement.

U

Ulcer: Open sore or lesion on skin or mucous membranes.

Ulna: Smaller lower arm bone.

Umbilical Cord: Cord with two arteries and one vein connecting the fetus to the placenta.

Ureter: Tube connecting the kidney to the bladder.

Urethra: Tube from the bladder to the outside.

Urethritis: Inflammation of the urethra.

Urinary Tract Infection (UTI): Infection of the urethra, bladder, and/or ureters.

Urticaria: Hives.

Urushiol: Resinous oil found in poison ivy, poison oak, and poison sumac that causes an allergic reaction.

Uterus: Organ of the female reproductive system that supports a fetus.

V

Vasoconstriction: A narrowing of blood vessels.

Vasodilation: A widening of blood vessels.

Vasogenic: Originating in the vessels.

Vein: Vessel carrying blood toward the heart.

Venule: Small vein.

Vertigo: Dizziness caused by a disturbance in equilibrium.

Virus: Microorganism that depends on another organism's cells as a host for replication.

X

Xiphoid Process: Flexible, cartilaginous protuberance at the lower end of the sternum.

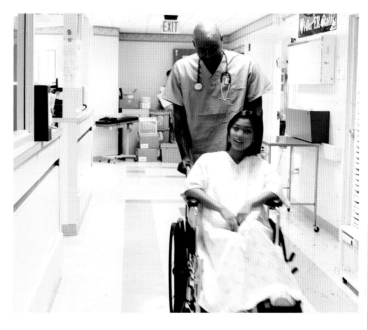

INDEX

INDEX

INDEX

INDEX